Disorders of Sex Development

A JOHNS HOPKINS PRESS HEALTH BOOK

disorders of sex development

A Guide for PARENTS *and* PHYSICIANS

Amy B. Wisniewski, Ph.D.

Steven D. Chernausek, M.D.

Bradley P. Kropp, M.D.

The Johns Hopkins University Press

Baltimore

A portion of the proceeds from this book funds support groups for families and patients with disorders of sex development.

Note to the reader: This book describes disorders of sex development in children in general. It was not written about your child. The information in this book should by no means be considered a substitute for the advice of qualified medical professionals. The services of competent professionals should be obtained whenever medical or other specific advice is needed.

Printed in the United States of America on acid-free paper
9 8 7 6 5 4 3 2 1

The Johns Hopkins University Press
2715 North Charles Street
Baltimore, Maryland 21218-4363
www.press.jhu.edu

Library of Congress Cataloging-in-Publication Data

Wisniewski, Amy B.
Disorders of sex development : a guide for parents and physicians / Amy B. Wisniewski, Steven D. Chernausek, and Bradley P. Kropp.
p. cm. — (A Johns Hopkins Press health book)
Includes index.
ISBN-13: 978-1-4214-0501-8 (hdbk. : alk. paper)
ISBN-13: 978-1-4214-0502-5 (pbk. : alk. paper)
ISBN-13: 978-1-4214-0540-7 (electronic)
ISBN-10: 1-4214-0501-6 (hdbk. : alk. paper)
ISBN-10: 1-4214-0502-4 (pbk. : alk. paper)
ISBN-10: 1-4214-0540-7 (electronic)
1. Sex differentiation disorders—Popular works. 2. Sex disorders—Popular works. 3. Generative organs—Growth—Diseases—Popular works. I. Chernausek, Steven D. II. Kropp, Bradley P. III. Title.
RC883.5.S47W57 2012
616.6′94—dc23 2011029766

A catalog record for this book is available from the British Library.

All figures are by Michelle Davis.

Special discounts are available for bulk purchases of this book. For more information, please contact Special Sales at 410-516-6936 or specialsales@press.jhu.edu.

The Johns Hopkins University Press uses environmentally friendly book materials, including recycled text paper that is composed of at least 30 percent post-consumer waste, whenever possible.

To London and her family,
and to all of the patients and families in the SUCCEED Clinic.
Thank you for teaching us every day.

Contents

Preface

This book is for people with disorders of sex development (DSD) and their parents and physicians. We decided to write this book because we know that there is not much information about DSD for the general public. We combined our roles as physicians, educators, and researchers to produce a resource that would inform parents, people with DSD, and their health care teams about DSD conditions as well as about options for treatments and outcomes. Here, we have attempted to assemble practical information about DSD so that readers can become more knowledgeable about and feel more confident in discussing DSD.

This book explains what DSD is, how it is diagnosed, and which laboratory and imaging tests are relied upon to establish a diagnosis. You may read the entire book from beginning to end for a more global understanding of DSD, or you may want to focus on individual chapters to answer specific questions. The book begins by discussing DSD in newborns, but it also considers questions that arise as a child with DSD matures, so readers may find it helpful to return periodically to the book over time. Key questions covered are listed at the beginning of each chapter.

At first, you might not be familiar with such medical terms as Müllerian inhibiting substance and 46,XX. We walk you through these terms, step by step. Soon you will have the information and the words you need to discuss your child's individual situation and get the most benefit from your interactions with health care professionals.

Certain aspects of care for people with DSD are controversial, such as surgery and experimental treatments. Although we do not have all the answers about whether these options are in the best interest of patients, and particularly whether they are right for *your* child, we have tried to present a balanced view so readers can make informed decisions. We have also included suggestions about how to talk about DSD with other family members and with doctors, as well as how to meet other people who have DSD to share information and support. Knowledge empowers individuals.

Though we occasionally make specific recommendations for the management of DSD, the purpose of this book is educating and encouraging everyone, not defining optimal treatments for any specific individual. Every person with DSD has aspects of his or her condition that need an individualized approach, and care for people who have DSD continues to evolve. Readers are therefore advised to consult the most current information available from health care professionals and other sources when making decisions about treatment.

Our hope is that this book will help parents and physicians make it possible for children with DSD to lead the ordinary—and extraordinary—lives that they deserve. For individuals with DSD, we hope that this book acts as a resource throughout life.

Disorders of Sex Development

• 1 •

An Introduction to DSD

Key Questions

What is DSD?
How are children with DSD identified?
Did I cause my child to have DSD?
Is my child a boy or a girl?
Will my child grow up to be healthy and happy?

A "disorder of sex development," or DSD, refers to a medical condition in which there is disagreement between a person's genetic sex (that is, chromosomes) and the appearance of their external or internal reproductive structures. For example, a child with DSD may have a female genetic sex, but the genital structures appear male-like or masculinized. Some people believe that the term "disorders" of sex development connotes sickness; therefore, the term "differences" in sex development may be preferred when talking about DSD.

Most people affected by DSD grow up to lead healthy, happy lives. We believe that the best predictors of health and happiness for people with DSD are (1) a meaningful understanding of their medical condition and (2) support from friends and loved ones. People with DSD and their families benefit from education and advice from an experienced team of professionals.

We wrote this book for people with DSD, their parents and other family members, and medical professionals. Reading this book will help you understand DSD and provide a framework that will enable you and your child to deal with many of the aspects of having a DSD.

The diagnosis of DSD can be frightening. But you can lessen your fear with a better understanding of what brought about a particular DSD in the first place and what is really involved in having a DSD. The purpose of this chapter is to explain the biology behind DSD and to provide basic information about the general development of affected children. We start with an explanation of the typical sequence of events that takes place as male and female babies develop in the womb. This information will help you understand how your child's DSD came about and will allow you to better support your child as he or she grows from infancy through adulthood.

For most parents, the diagnosis of DSD comes as a surprise soon after the delivery of their baby. Common questions families and friends ask when they are told their baby has a DSD include *What is DSD? How is DSD identified? Did we do something to cause our child's DSD? Is my baby a boy or a girl? Will my child grow up to be normal and happy?* We begin by considering each of these questions.

What Is DSD?

A disorder of sex development is a medical condition in which the step-by-step development of reproductive structures that usually occurs early in pregnancy has been interrupted or altered. Many types of DSD are not life-threatening, but some do carry the serious risk of endangering life. We provide information on the risks in certain types of DSD in chapter 5.

Because the term "DSD" refers to a wide variety of medical conditions that differ significantly in their treatment and outcomes, people with one type of DSD may have much—or little—in common with those who are affected by another type. For many reasons, you want to know, when possible, what kind of DSD your child has. This information allows you to focus on information and medical advice that is relevant to your child's situation. For example, when you search on the Internet, you will be able to look for information about DSD that applies specifically to what your family is experiencing. Chapters 2 and 3 explain the different types of DSD that occur and the medical tests used to diagnose them.

To understand how DSD happens, let us first consider the process of typical sex determination and differentiation. In other words, why do some fetuses grow into girls while others grow into boys when developing in their mother's womb? At the start of gestation, babies do not yet exhibit a sex; we refer to these babies as being "sex neutral." All babies are capable of becoming girls or boys, but, very early in pregnancy, genetic and hormonal events usually occur that support either female or male development.

Sex Determination

Why do some babies become female while others become male? We use the term "sex determination" to describe the first steps that determine whether a child will develop into a male or female. Remember that all babies start with both male and female parts, whether or not they have DSD. For these children, certain things happen to make the parts of one sex develop fully while the other structures remain undeveloped. Usually, the sex chromosomes are the first signal as to which developmental plan the growing baby's body will follow. Mothers typically contribute an X chromosome, while fathers typically contribute an X or a Y chromosome to their child (figure 1.1). The end result is a baby who has a pair of sex chromosomes that are either XX (genetic female) or XY (genetic male). Babies who do not possess a Y chromosome usually follow a female path as they grow. In contrast, babies who possess a Y chromosome usually follow a male path.

Sex Differentiation

We use the term "sex differentiation" to describe events that occur after sex determination that lead to a fully formed male or

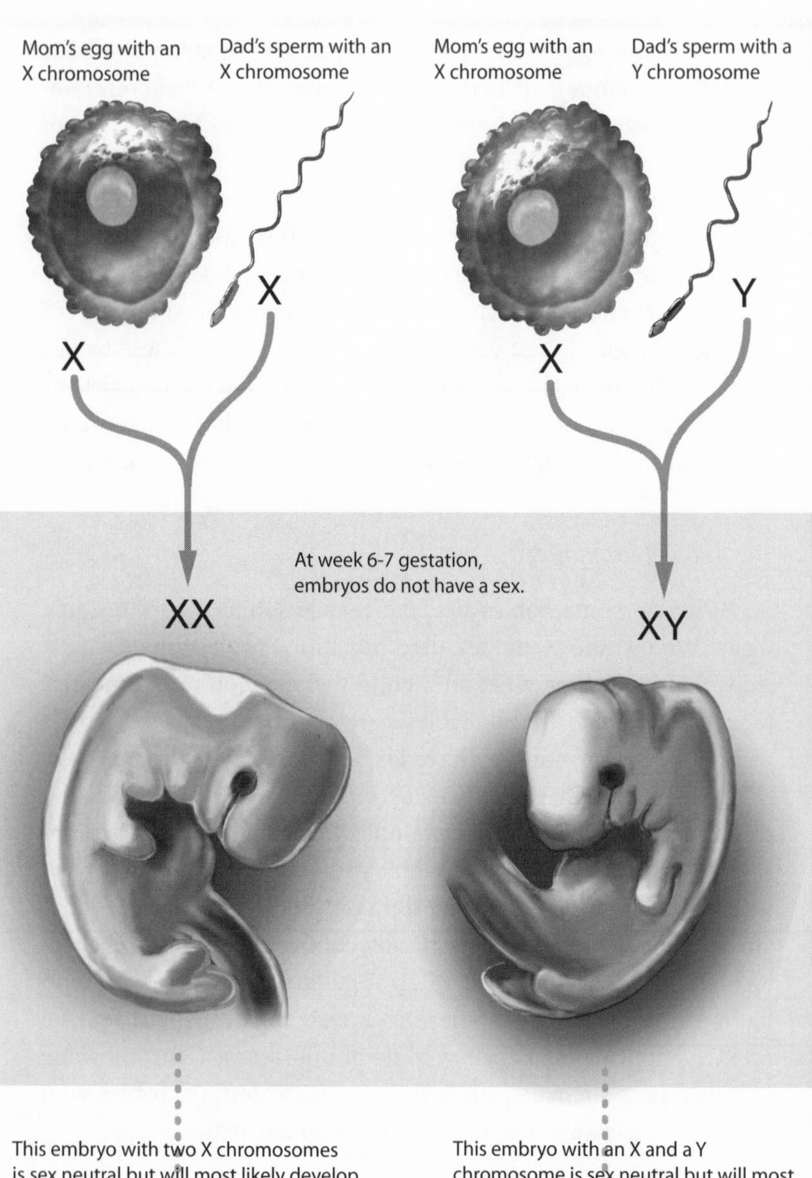

This embryo with two X chromosomes is sex neutral but will most likely develop into a female.

This embryo with an X and a Y chromosome is sex neutral but will most likely develop into a male.

♀

♂

female child at birth. Once the sex chromosomes "determine" a particular path of development, the sex-neutral baby develops either female or male anatomy. For either sex to develop, hormones need to act on anatomical structures at precise stages of development. These hormones are normally produced by the gonads: ovaries in females and testes in males. A person's gonadal sex refers to whether they develop ovaries or testes. Let's consider how a developing baby girl forms ovaries, while a developing baby boy forms testes.

Gonadal Development

A baby who possesses a female set of sex chromosomes (two X chromosomes, one from mom and one from dad) usually grows ovaries from tissue that exists in an earlier, less developed stage. Scientists have not yet completely figured out how the early tissue differentiates into ovaries in the presence of two X chromosomes. We only know that most people who are genetically female develop ovaries during the first 8 weeks of growth in the womb (figure 1.2). A baby who possesses a male set of chromosomes (an X from mom and a Y from dad) usually grows testes from early sex-neutral tissue.

We do have a good scientific understanding of how testicular development occurs. A gene found on the Y chromosome, called *SRY*, signals sex-neutral tissue to develop into a pair of testes (figure 1.2). If the *SRY* gene is missing or does not work, then the baby will not grow healthy testes despite having a male genetic sex (XY). Conversely, if a baby who is genetically female (XX) possesses the *SRY* gene on any chromosome (this can happen by accidental

---

(*Opposite*) Figure 1.1. The beginning of sex determination.
The first step in sex determination involves the egg, which has one X chromosome, being fertilized by a sperm that carries either an X or a Y chromosome. The fertilized egg then has either two Xs (female typical) or an X and Y (male typical). Even so, all fetuses start off sex neutral and then develop into girls or boys as they grow in the womb.

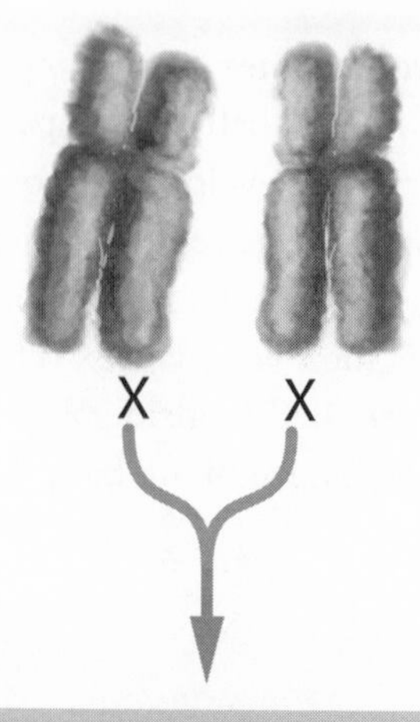

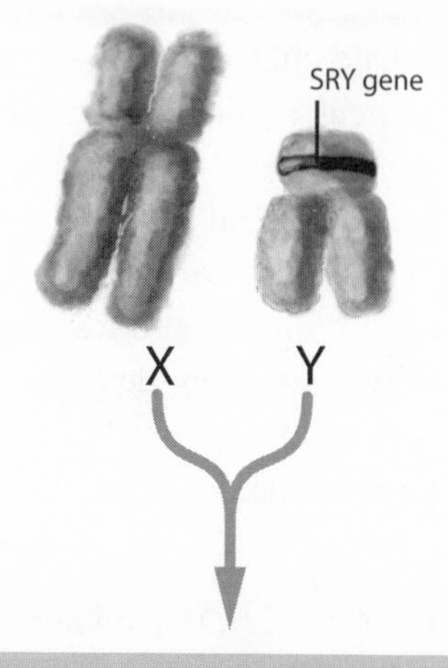

8 week (gestational age) embryo
with NO SRY gene

8 week (gestational age) embryo
with the SRY gene

ovary

In the absence of *SRY,*
ovaries develop from
sex-neutral gonadal tissue.

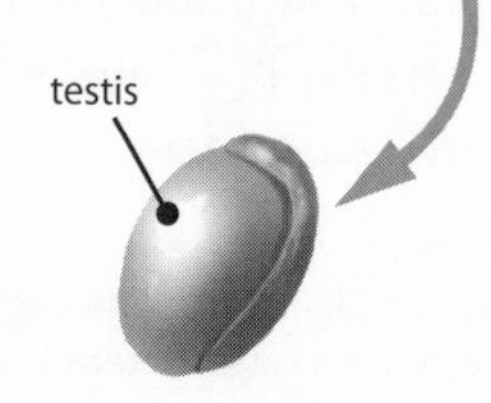

In the presence of *SRY*,
testes develop from
sex-neutral gonadal tissue.

rearrangement of genes), then testes will develop instead of ovaries. In other words, the absence or presence of the *SRY* gene, and not chromosomal sex per se, determines whether testes develop. The important role that this gene plays in gonadal differentiation explains why doctors often test for its presence or absence at a very early point when evaluating a child with DSD. This type of testing is explained further in chapter 3.

Gonadal Hormones

Developing ovaries and testes differ not only in appearance but also in how they work. For the most part, young ovaries make no hormones needed for early sex differentiation. In contrast, young testes produce significant amounts of two important hormones: testosterone and Müllerian inhibiting substance (MIS). You will learn more about Müllerian ducts and their role in the development of genitalia in the next section. The production of *both* testosterone and MIS is needed for a baby to develop male reproductive anatomy. In the *absence* of testosterone and MIS, female anatomy is formed even when a Y chromosome is present. This applies to the internal structures needed for future fertility (such as a uterus and fallopian tubes), as well as the external genital structures.

Development of Internal Sex Ducts

The sex ducts are the starting material for the internal reproductive structures. All babies, regardless of their genetic sex (XX or XY), have *both* female and male internal sex ducts early in devel-

---

(*Opposite*) Figure 1.2. Gonadal differentiation.
Before the fetus reaches the gestational age of 8 weeks, gonadal tissue has the potential to develop into either ovaries or testes and is considered sex neutral. The absence or presence of the *SRY* gene, usually located on the Y chromosome, determines whether this tissue will differentiate into ovaries (when *SRY* is absent) or testes (when *SRY* is present).

opment when sex neutral. Female ducts, called Müllerian ducts, develop into all of the internal reproductive structures of women (except for the ovaries, which develop from the early, sex-neutral gonadal tissue). These female ducts grow because, without testes, there is no MIS to block their development. A baby who is not exposed to MIS in the womb forms the following internal structures: the upper end of the vagina, the cervix, the uterus, and the fallopian tubes. Male ducts, called Wolffian ducts, grow into the epididymides, the vas deferentia, and the seminal vesicles, which are the internal reproductive structures of men that are needed for sperm to leave the body. These male ducts develop in response to the hormone testosterone. When Wolffian ducts are exposed to high levels of testosterone, a baby forms the internal structures shown in figure 1.3.

Let's review typical female development up to this point. First, a baby is formed with a female chromosomal sex (XX) because each parent contributes an X chromosome. Because the *SRY* gene is usually located on the Y chromosome, the baby lacks this gene. Ovaries develop from early tissue that is sex neutral. Because ovaries do not produce the hormone MIS, the Müllerian (female) ducts grow into the internal structures needed for a woman to carry a pregnancy. Because ovaries do not make testosterone, the Wolffian (male) ducts do not develop. In summary, we have a genetically female (XX) baby with female gonads (ovaries) and internal female

---

(*Opposite*) Figure 1.3. Formation of internal reproductive structures. Fetal ovaries make negligible amounts of testosterone and Müllerian inhibiting substance (MIS), but fetal testes produce significant amounts of both hormones. The presence or absence of these hormones influences development of the internal sex ducts, which fall into two categories. Müllerian ducts (forerunners of the uterus, cervix, fallopian tubes, and upper portion of the vagina) are found in male and female fetuses but typically disappear in boy fetuses when the fetal testes make MIS. Wolffian ducts (from which vas deferentia, epididymides, prostate gland, and seminal vesicles arise) are likewise found in all fetuses but typically disappear in girl fetuses because they have no testes to produce testosterone. Thus it is the presence or absence of testosterone and MIS that determine whether the fetus will develop male or female internal reproductive anatomy.

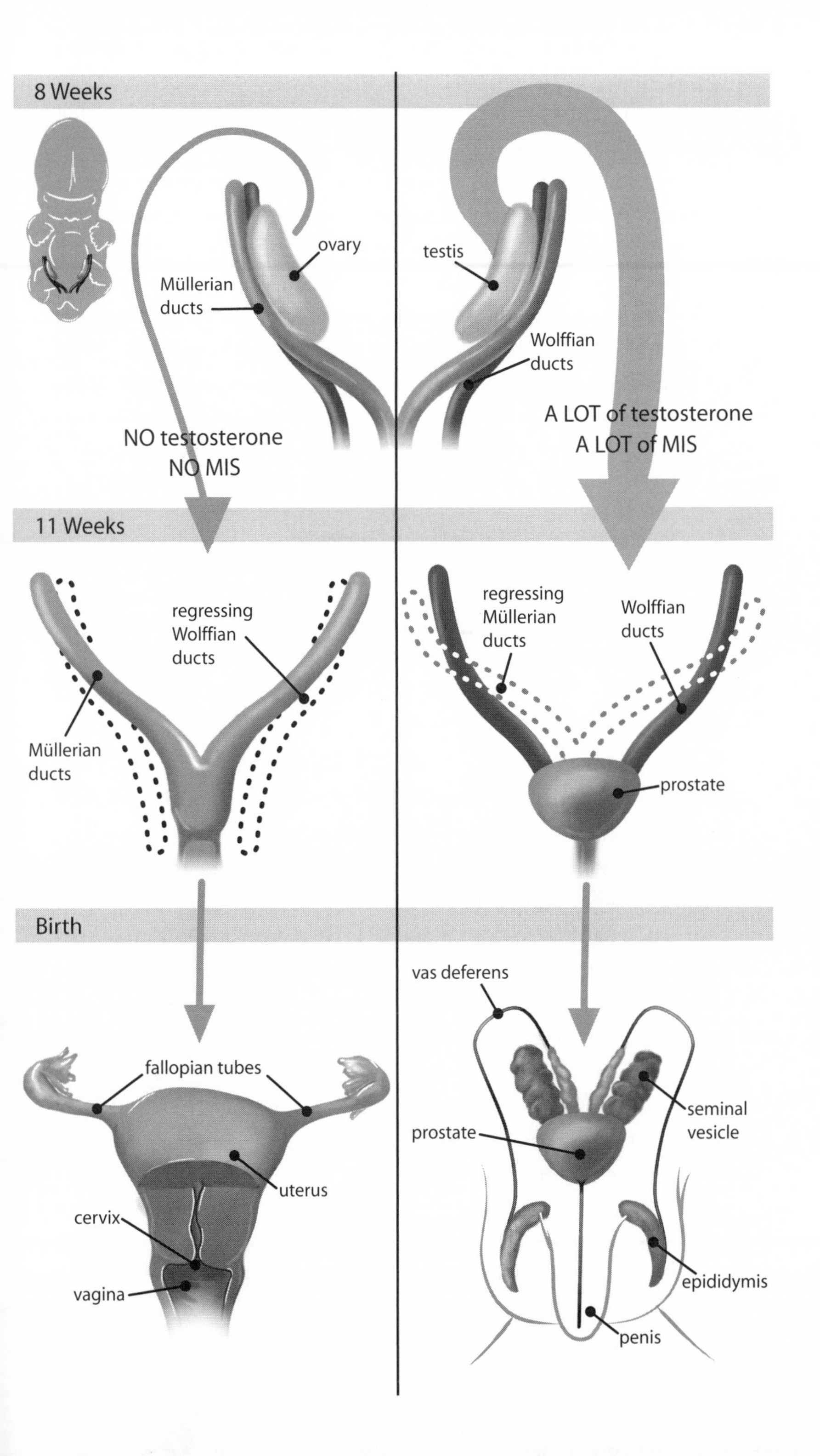
8 Weeks
ovary
Müllerian
ducts
testis
Wolffian
ducts
NO testosterone
NO MIS
A LOT of testosterone
A LOT of MIS
11 Weeks
regressing
Wolffian
ducts
Müllerian
ducts
regressing
Müllerian
ducts
Wolffian
ducts
prostate
Birth
fallopian tubes
uterus
cervix
vagina
vas deferens
seminal
vesicle
prostate
epididymis
penis

(Müllerian) reproductive structures and no accompanying internal male (Wolffian) reproductive structures.

Let us also review typical male development. A baby will have a male chromosomal sex if mom contributes an X chromosome and dad contributes a Y chromosome. Because the Y chromosome encodes the *SRY* gene, the baby grows testes from its sex-neutral tissue. The testes produce testosterone and MIS. The MIS inhibits the Müllerian (female) internal ducts, and testosterone promotes growth of the Wolffian (male) internal ducts. The result is a genetically male (XY) baby with male gonads (testes) and internal male reproductive structures with no accompanying female internal ducts.

Development of the External Genitalia

Up to this point, we have considered how a female or male typically develops a chromosomal sex, gonadal sex, and internal reproductive parts. For most of us, none of these aspects of sex are obvious at birth. What is announced at birth is delivery room sex—or the type of external genitalia a newborn exhibits (that is, labia, clitoris, and vaginal opening collectively referred to as the vulva for girls and penis and scrotum for boys). Growth of the external genitalia is the final part of sex differentiation to consider.

A baby who does not make a by-product of the hormone testosterone called dihydrotestosterone (DHT) will grow a vulva. In contrast, a baby who does make DHT will grow a penis and scrotum (see figure 1.4). DHT is made in our bodies when an enzyme called 5α-reductase is available. This enzyme changes testosterone to DHT. From the earlier description of the development of the gonads and sex ducts, it is clear that more is involved with growing into a female or a male than simply chromosomal sex (XX or XY). The same is true for the developing external genitalia. This is why some children with a male chromosomal sex (XY) appear female, while others with a female chromosomal sex (XX) appear male. Some children, regardless of their chromosomal sex, are born with external genitalia that appear neither obviously male nor female. When this happens, we say these children have ambiguous genitalia.

How Are Children with DSD Identified?

Many children affected by DSD are identified at birth because they are born with ambiguous external genitalia. Ambiguous external genitalia may include a phallic structure that is smaller than a penis but larger than a clitoris, and labia-like structures that are partially fused to look somewhat like a scrotum. Other children affected by DSD are identified when it is noted that either their chromosomal sex or gonadal sex does not match their external genital sex. This may occur when a mother undergoes prenatal tests to determine the genetic sex of her baby and the results do not match what is observed in the delivery room.

When a child is born with genital ambiguity, we generally think of one of two common scenarios. In one scenario, the child is chromosomally female (XX) with masculinized external genitalia (an enlarged clitoris and labial fusion) due to excess exposure to DHT during life in the womb. In the other scenario, the child is chromosomally male (XY) with undermasculinized external genitalia (a small penis and unfused scrotum) due to insufficient DHT production or action.

Less commonly, DSD is identified later in life. For example, children with complete androgen insensitivity syndrome (CAIS, discussed in chapter 2) are frequently diagnosed when testes are found in the groin of a young girl during a routine physical examination or hernia repair. Chapter 2 describes different types of DSD in more detail and chapter 3 explains how these conditions are identified and diagnosed.

Did I Cause My Child to Have DSD?

Many parents, upon learning that their child is affected by DSD, wonder if they did something to cause the condition. Some drugs

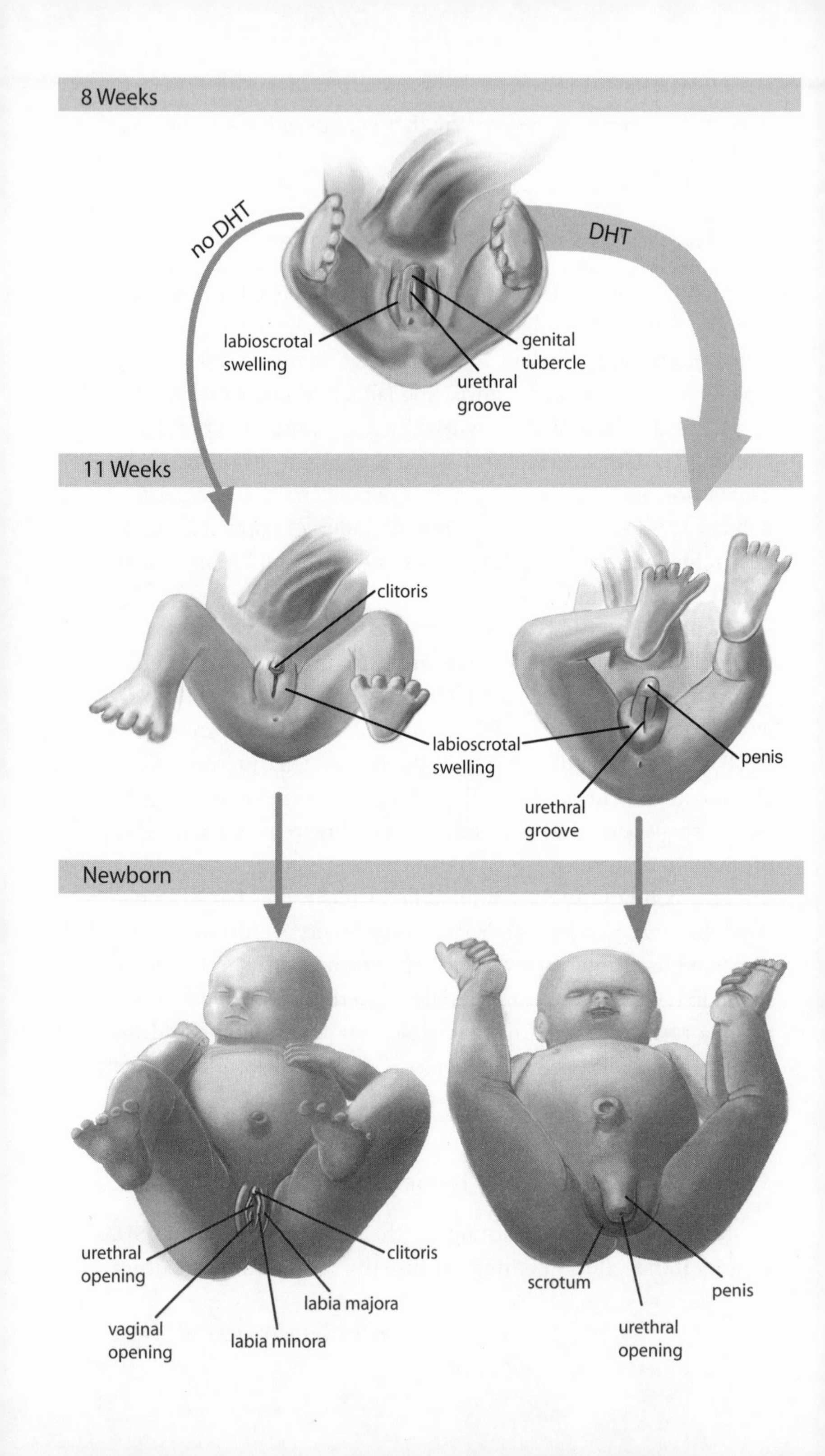
8 Weeks
no DHT
DHT
labioscrotal swelling
genital tubercle
urethral groove
11 Weeks
clitoris
labioscrotal swelling
penis
urethral groove
Newborn
urethral opening
clitoris
labia majora
vaginal opening
labia minora
scrotum
penis
urethral opening

administered to pregnant women in the past, such as diethylstilbesterol (DES) and progesterone, caused ambiguous genitalia in babies. These drugs are no longer given during pregnancy. The best scientific knowledge at this time tells us that parents do not usually cause their children to be affected by DSD as a result of medication use or lifestyle habits. If parents use medications as directed by their doctors, this will not cause their child to have DSD. If parents eat certain types of food, this will not cause their child to have DSD. If parents exercise or don't exercise, this will not cause their child to have DSD. These medical conditions generally occur as a result of new or inherited genetic signals that alter sex determination or differentiation. Just as your child did not choose the genes she or he inherited from you, you did not choose the genes that you passed on to your child. Therefore, even if your child's DSD is a result of a genetic mutation inherited from you, you did not choose for your child to have DSD. If you are planning future pregnancies, you may want to consult a genetic counselor who can help families determine the likelihood that future children might also be affected by DSD.

It is normal for parents to feel guilt when their child is born with a medical condition. Unlike medical problems like asthma that are caused by secondhand smoke exposure or developmental delay due to fetal alcohol exposure, DSD does not occur because parents did anything wrong during either pregnancy or child rearing. The

---

(*Opposite*) Figure 1.4. Development of the external genitals.
At 8 weeks (*top*) the fetus's external genitals are sex neutral, but they can go on to form female-typical structures (*left*) or male-typical structures (*right*) depending on hormone exposure. In fetal development, the absence of a by-product of testosterone called dihydrotestosterone (DHT) results in female external genitalia, and the presence of DHT results in the growth of male external genitalia. In the *absence* of DHT, the genital tubercle stays small and forms a clitoris. In addition, the urethral groove develops into a urinary opening that is located on the perineum, as is typical for females. Finally, the labioscrotal swellings go on to form the labia. In the *presence* of DHT the genital tubercle grows into a penis, the urethral fold develops so that the urinary opening is at the tip of the penis, and the labioscrotal swellings fuse to make the scrotum.

very fact that you are taking the time to read this book and educate yourself about your child's health shows your commitment to good parenting and your wish to provide the best for your child.

Is My Child a Boy or a Girl?

Often there is a question about a child's sex when a DSD is identified. Of the many experiences associated with DSD, this is perhaps one of the most difficult for new parents. Children have a clearly identified sex: female or male. Your child is no different: she or he has a sex too. One of the services that your medical team can provide is help in determining the best gender of rearing for your baby. Factors considered when recommending a gender include what is known about the long-term behavioral development of people with specific types of DSD, the child's reproductive anatomy, and the child's potential for future fertility and sexual function. This information is discussed in greater detail in chapter 4. For older children who have already been assigned a gender, the health care team can help by providing education and support about why that decision was made.

Will My Child Grow up to Be Healthy and Happy?

One of the joys of parenting is to watch an infant grow into a child and then an adult. Some parts of your child's personality and thoughts will very likely be consistent with those of other members of your family. Other aspects of your child will assuredly be unique. Nobody (including the authors of this book) can predict with complete accuracy how any child will ultimately grow up, whether or not they are affected by DSD. We can, however, offer some information about development that parents might expect to observe in their child who has a DSD. One of these is the likelihood that your child will accept his or her gender of rearing. By this we mean that your child will continue to live as the gender that he or she was reared because he or she accepts and identifies with that gender.

When gender assignment takes into consideration the type of DSD and outcome data for psychological development, most people are happy with the decisions made by their parents and physicians. As we mentioned earlier, educating yourself and your child about DSD increases the likelihood that this will happen for your child.

• *Chapter Summary* •

It is understandable for parents to experience concern, guilt, and possibly even anger when they learn that their baby is affected by DSD. It is important to know how DSD happens and realize that parents did nothing to purposely cause this condition in their child. To increase the likelihood that their child will lead a happy and healthy life, parents can stay informed about their child's health and find an experienced medical team that will include the family in making decisions concerning their child's care and support.

One of these decisions may be choosing the best gender of rearing for a child. To make this decision, what is known about psychological development in people with specific types of DSD needs to be considered. Once this and other decisions are made, it is time for your family to welcome and enjoy your new baby.

• 2 •

What Type of DSD Does My Child Have?

Key Questions

What is 46,XX DSD?
What is 46,XY DSD?
What other types of DSD are there?

Most parents find out that their child has a DSD when their baby is born with ambiguous genitalia. Understandably, from the moment they see or hear about their baby's condition, parents want to know what type of DSD the baby has, what the baby's sex is, and what treatment is recommended for their baby. But at the moment the baby is born it is likely that the answers to these questions aren't known. Only laboratory testing and further evaluation will provide answers.

The uncertainty that comes with having to wait for results is often frustrating to parents, because they naturally wish for immediate answers to questions concerning their child's health. This chapter explains the general categories of DSD so that, when the child's DSD has been defined, parents will know more about the child's condition. Chapter 3 describes the tests used to identify which type of DSD applies to your child. Taken together, the information from chapters 2 and 3 will help you feel more comfortable that you are making good decisions about your child's condition and care.

DSD refers to a wide array of medical conditions in which there is a discrepancy between a person's genetic sex (that is, chromosomes) and the appearance of their external or internal reproductive structures. For simplicity, we discuss DSD as being composed of three major categories: (1) 46,XX DSD, (2) 46,XY DSD, and (3) other types of DSD. More medical information is currently available about some types of DSD than others. We encourage you to consider all available information as you work with your child's health care team to develop the best plan for your son's or daughter's support and treatment.

What Is 46,XX DSD?

The term "46,XX DSD" is used to describe children who possess the usual total number of chromosomes (46) including two X chromosomes (female), but whose internal sex ducts or external genital structures do not develop in the typical female manner. For example, a baby born with 46,XX DSD may have a uterus and fallopian tubes but may also have external genital structures that are male-like, or masculine—such as an enlarged clitoris that resembles a penis or fused labia that look like a scrotum. In this case, because the genetic sex (46,XX) matches the internal sex ducts (uterus and fallopian tubes) but not the external genitals (enlarged clitoris and fused labia), we say that this baby has 46,XX DSD.

In chapter 1 we explained that the external genitalia differentiate depending on whether or not the hormone DHT is present before birth. This differentiation occurs regardless of the baby's genetic or gonadal sex. (Recall that gonadal sex refers to whether a person has developed ovaries or testes.) When DHT is absent, female external genitalia (a clitoris and labia) develop. When DHT is present in sufficient amounts, the external genitalia will tend to masculinize resulting in an enlarged clitoris and fused labia (figure 2.1), despite the baby's genetic sex. DHT causes the female baby's clitoris to grow bigger and the urinary opening (called the "urethral meatus") to move toward the tip. When exposed to DHT,

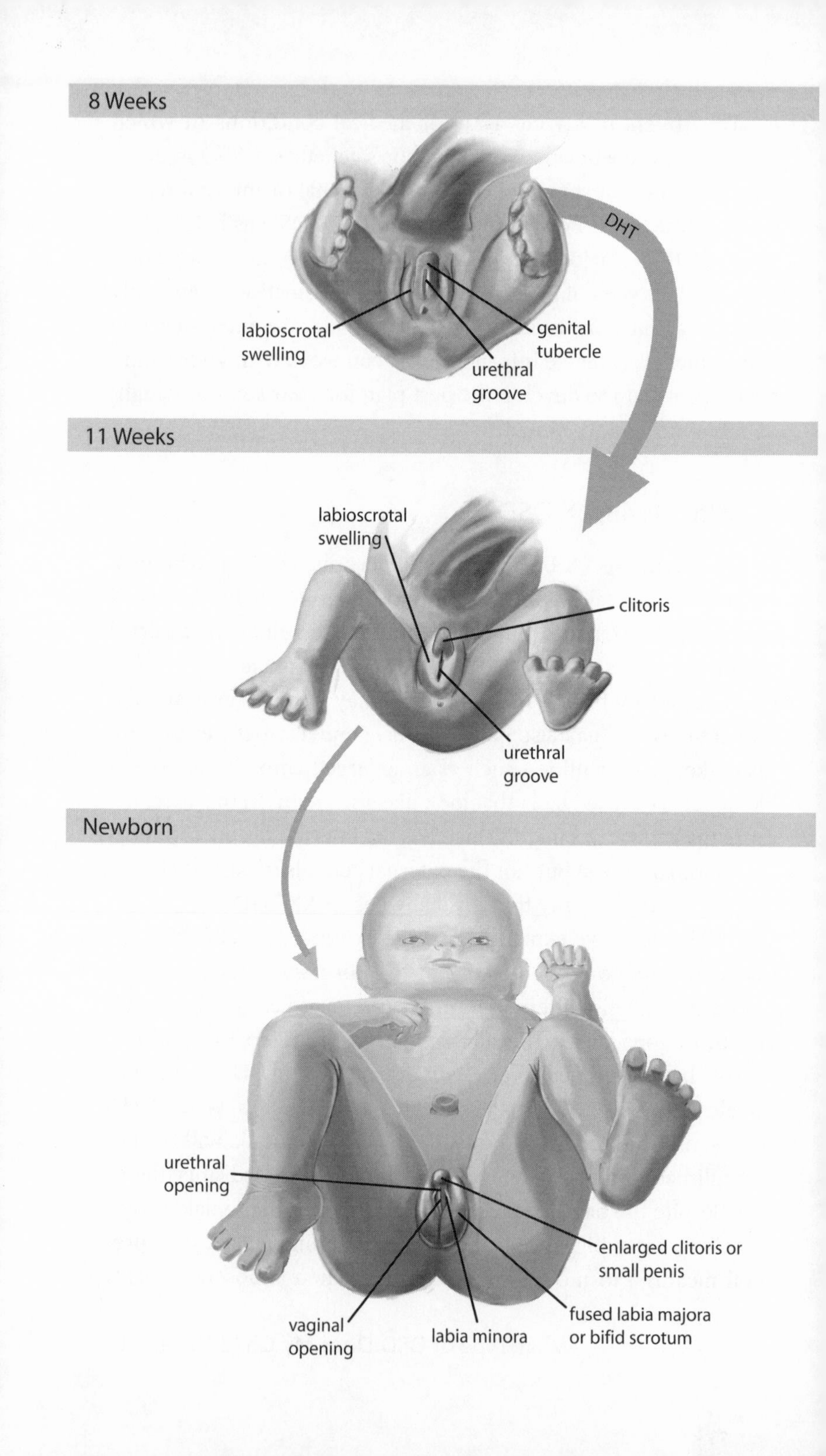
8 Weeks
DHT
labioscrotal swelling
genital tubercle
urethral groove
11 Weeks
labioscrotal swelling
clitoris
urethral groove
Newborn
urethral opening
enlarged clitoris or small penis
fused labia majora or bifid scrotum
vaginal opening
labia minora

babies' labia fuse together to form a structure that resembles a scrotum.

If a baby's sex chromosomes and internal sex ducts are both typical of a female, we would expect this baby to have ovaries and not testes (chapter 3 explains how the sex of the internal sex ducts is confirmed). Why then would a baby with 46,XX who has female internal sex ducts and ovaries be born with masculinized external genitalia? Remember that DHT is the hormone that converts the female external genitalia to the masculine form. So we can assume that this baby was exposed to DHT prior to birth. There are several ways that this can happen. The most common way is a medical condition known as congenital adrenal hyperplasia (CAH) due to 21-hydroxylase, or 21-OH, deficiency in which a particular enzyme (21-hydroxylase) does not work properly, resulting in a hormonal imbalance. Because CAH due to 21-hydroxylase deficiency is the most common form of 46,XX DSD, we consider it first.

Congenital Adrenal Hyperplasia and 21-Hydrolase Deficiency

Most people are born with two adrenal glands located just above the kidneys. The outer portion of these glands, known as the cortex, produces hormones important for maintaining salt balance

---

(*Opposite*) Figure 2.1. DSD with ambiguous genitalia.
This child has had some exposure to dihydrotestosterone (DHT) but not enough to complete the formation of a typical male penis and scrotum. The physical appearance shown here is characteristic for 46,XX DSD—a disorder of sex development involving a typical chromosome count of 46 and two X chromosomes but atypical female genitalia. In the presence of DHT, the genital tubercle enlarges to resemble a large clitoris or a small penis and the labioscrotal swellings fuse to look like a scrotum, but the opening for the passage of urine is on the perineum where the labia are only partially fused. Sometimes there is a common opening to both the urethra and vagina, called a "urogenital sinus." However, the appearance of the external genitals alone does not tell us whether this child has 46,XY DSD or 46,XX DSD. Many children with 46,XY DSD have the same external anatomy as children with 46,XX DSD, so chromosome testing and other studies are needed to complete the assessment.

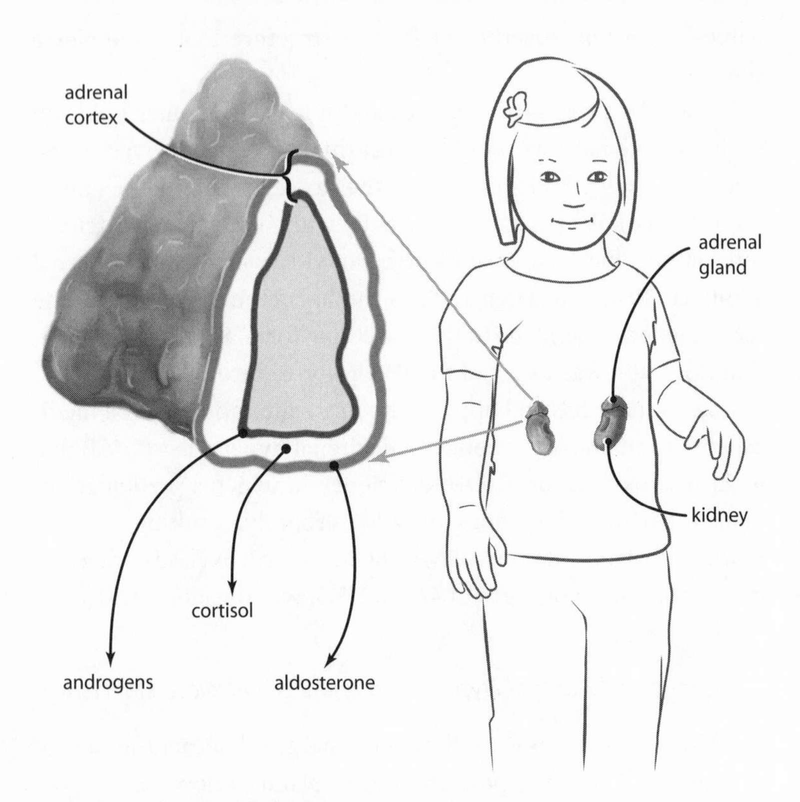

Figure 2.2. The adrenal glands.
The outer portion of the adrenal gland, known as the cortex, produces hormones important for maintaining salt balance (aldosterone), responding to stress (cortisol), and sex development (androgens, including testosterone). When the glands do not produce the proper balance of hormones while a baby is in the womb, as is the case with CAH due to 21-hydroxylase (21-OH) deficiency, it can affect the development of the external genitalia in girls.

(aldosterone), responding to stress (cortisol), and sex development (testosterone, which is then converted to DHT in the genital tissues; figure 2.2). In CAH due to 21-hydroxylase deficiency, the fetus's adrenal glands lack the ability to make cortisol (and usually aldosterone as well), but there is no problem with testosterone production. Babies with this form of CAH try to overcome their inability to make cortisol by producing large amounts of the hormones needed to produce cortisol. These hormones rise to very high levels and are then changed by the adrenal glands into testosterone, which is then secreted into the bloodstream. This testosterone from the adrenals is then converted to DHT, causing the external genitals of affected girls to masculinize (figure 2.3) during fetal development.

For some girls, enough DHT is produced to cause the clitoris to enlarge and the labia to fuse. Girls affected by CAH due to 21-hydroxylase deficiency are born with varying degrees of external genital masculinization (also referred to as ambiguous genitalia). The degree of masculinization reflects the severity of the 21-hydroxylase enzyme deficiency. Simply put, a greater degree of 21-hydroxylase deficiency results in greater masculinization of the external genitalia at birth. For girls with CAH, the degree of masculinization of their external genitalia at birth is graded according to the Prader scale (figure 2.4).

Boys are *supposed* to be exposed to DHT during early fetal development, so when a boy has 21-hydroxylase deficiency, his external genitalia look like those of boys who don't have CAH.

Our book focuses on DSD, and our discussion here is limited to the aspects of 21-hydroxylase deficiency that relate to DSD. But it's important to note that children with 21-hydroxylase deficiency, whether they are boys or girls, need to have their deficiencies of the hormones cortisol and aldosterone treated to survive and be healthy. There is much you need to know if your child has this type of congenital adrenal hyperplasia, and you can find excellent resources dedicated to teaching and supporting children and their parents about this condition in the reference section of this book.

CAH and 11β-Hydroxylase Deficiency

Being deficient in the enzyme 11β-hydroxylase also results in congenital adrenal hyperplasia and in ambiguous external genitalia in fetuses with female (XX) chromosomes. It is much less common than 21-hydroxylase deficiency. Babies with this condition

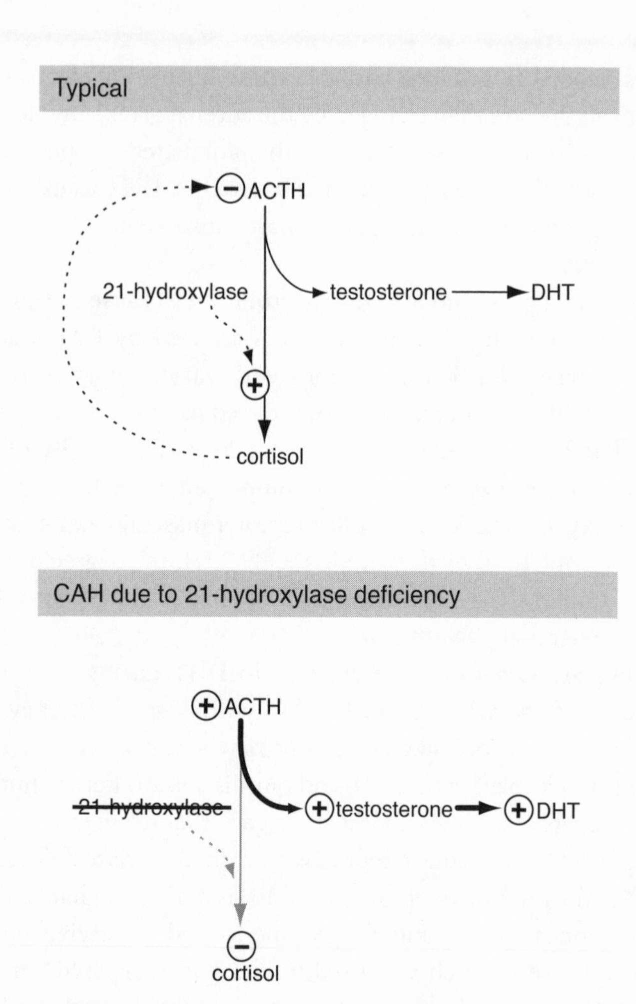

Figure 2.3. Adrenal function in CAH.
Typically the hypothalamus, pituitary, and adrenal glands work together to minimize adrenal production of testosterone and DHT while maintaining the right amount of cortisol in the bloodstream (*upper panel*). This happens because once cortisol is made, ACTH (a hormone from the pituitary that stimulates cortisol release) stops being produced until the body needs more stress hormone. In CAH due to 21-hydroxylase deficiency (*lower panel*), the fetus's adrenal glands lack the ability to make cortisol (and usually aldosterone) but can make testosterone and DHT. Because cortisol is absent, ACTH is never inhibited so it continues to stimulate adrenal androgen production in excess amounts. This hormonal environment causes the external genitals to be masculinized if the fetus is female (46,XX).

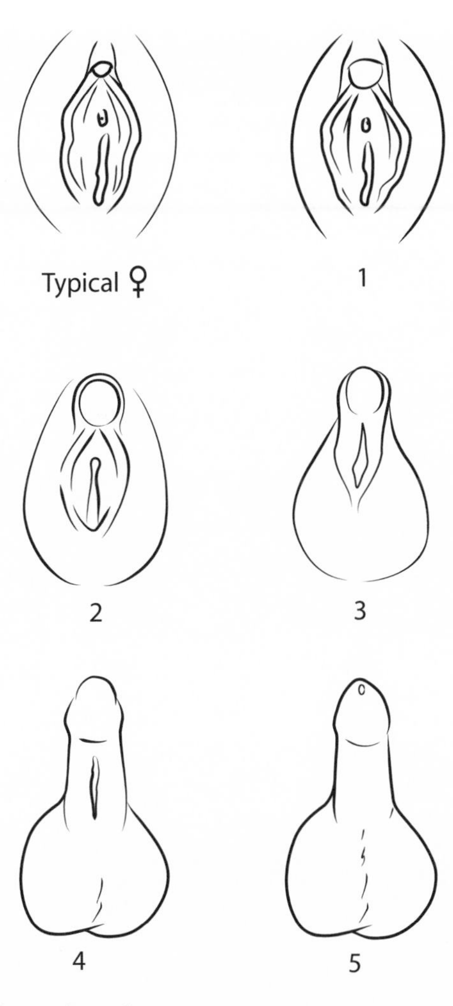

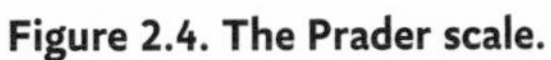
Figure 2.4. The Prader scale.

This scale is used to grade different degrees of masculinization of the external genitalia of girls with congenital adrenal hyperplasia (CAH), beginning with typical female genitalia (*upper left*) and progressing to typical male external genitalia (Prader 5, *lower right*). This scale does not reflect internal genitalia, which usually is the same as girls without CAH.

are also unable to make appropriate amounts of the hormone cortisol, and a build-up of DHT results (see figure 2.3). Similar to female babies with 21-hydroxylase deficiency, genetic females with 11β-hydroxylase deficiency possess ovaries and female internal sex ducts. An additional concern for these individuals is that they can develop high blood pressure.

Other Causes

Babies with 46,XX can develop DSD for reasons other than CAH. For example, if a mother has a hormone-producing tumor or if there are problems with the function of the placenta, the fetus may be exposed to DHT during early development in amounts sufficient to cause ambiguous external genitalia to form.

What Is 46,XY DSD?

The term "46,XY DSD" is used to describe a child with a 46,XY chromosome makeup whose internal or external reproductive structures did not develop fully in a manner typical for a male. For example, a child born with 46,XY DSD may possess male internal sex ducts (such as epididymides and vas deferentia) but have undermasculinized external genital anatomy. Undermasculinized external anatomy can include a very small phallus that looks more like a clitoris than a penis, an unfused scrotum that partially resembles labia, testes that have not dropped into the scrotum, and a urinary opening at the base of the phallus instead of at the tip (see figure 2.1). If the genetic sex (46,XY) matches the internal sex ducts (epididymides and vas deferentia) but not the external genital anatomy, the individual is said to have some type of a 46,XY DSD.

What caused this baby's 46,XY DSD to happen? Unlike 46,XX DSD, where the cause is usually CAH, reasons for developing 46,XY DSD are much more varied. To complicate matters further, in about half of all cases no clear cause for 46,XY DSD is ever identified. Despite these obstacles, we can generally attribute the situation to the inability either to produce or to respond to testicular hormones during fetal life.

Problems with Testicular Hormone Production

For male sex differentiation to proceed in the usual way, the testes need to make sufficient amounts of the hormones Müllerian inhibiting substance (MIS) and testosterone during the first 3 months of pregnancy. MIS is required to suppress female internal sex duct development. Testosterone is needed to promote male internal sex duct development. Furthermore, the testosterone must be converted to the potent hormone DHT, which then masculinizes the female-appearing external genitalia into a fully formed penis and scrotum. If a baby is unable to produce MIS, testosterone, or DHT in sufficient amounts to support male sex differentiation, a variety of types of DSD will occur. In some cases, the hormone deficiencies are incomplete and babies with a 46,XY chromosomal makeup are born with the following: (1) testes (because the *SRY* gene needed to form testes is present on the Y chromosome), (2) partial development of internal female sex ducts (because the testes did not produce sufficient MIS to completely suppress the development of these structures), (3) partial development of the internal male sex ducts (because the testes did not produce sufficient amounts of testosterone to completely support development of these structures), and (4) ambiguous external genitalia (because DHT was not produced in sufficient amounts to masculinize the external genital structures; figure 2.5). When testes are unable to produce sufficient amounts of hormones to support male sex differentiation, this is sometimes due to "partial gonadal dysgenesis." Chapter 3 discusses laboratory tests that can distinguish between the different types of 46,XY DSD.

Some babies with 46,XY DSD aren't able to make any testicular hormones at all (MIS, testosterone, or DHT), sometimes due to "complete gonadal dysgenesis." This can happen when testes do not form, possibly because the *SRY* gene on the Y chromosome was

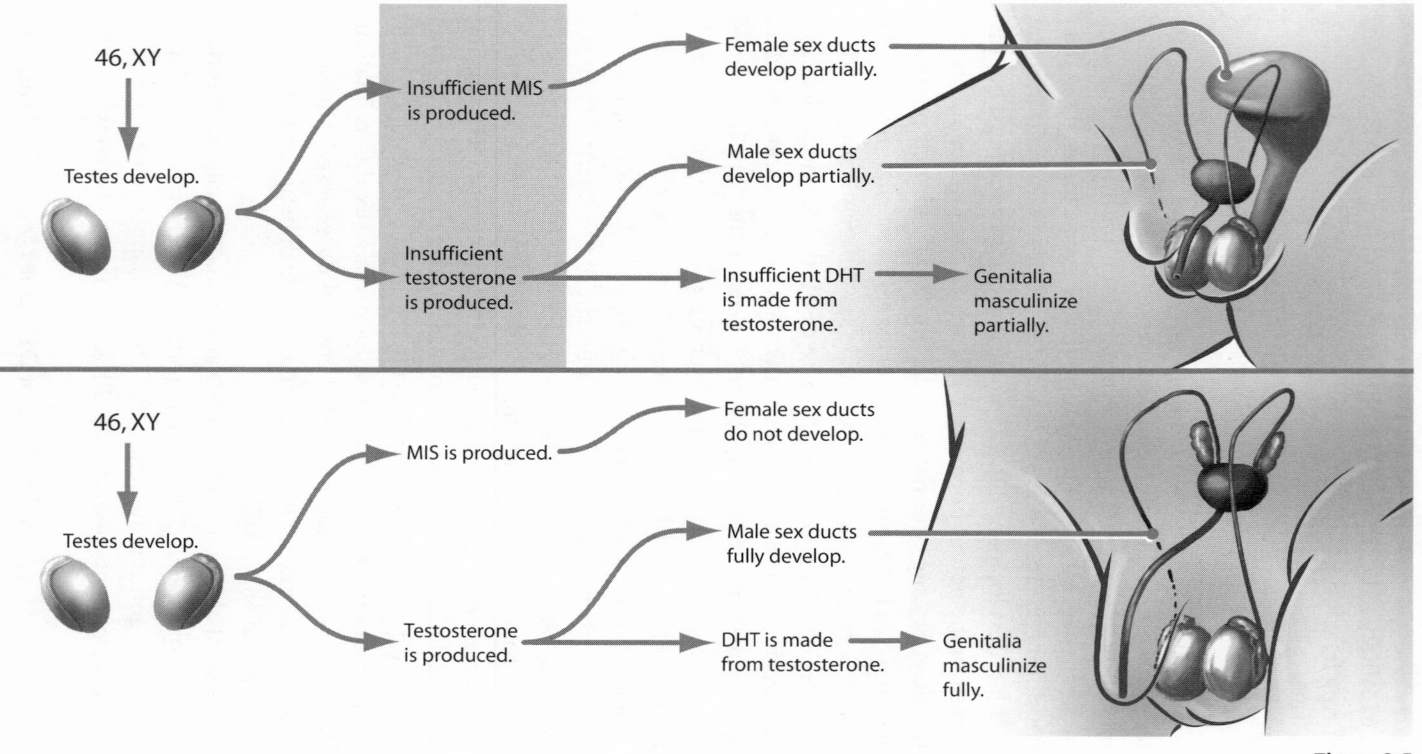
46, XY
Testes develop.
Insufficient MIS is produced.
Insufficient testosterone is produced.
Female sex ducts develop partially.
Male sex ducts develop partially.
Insufficient DHT is made from testosterone.
Genitalia masculinize partially.
46, XY
Testes develop.
MIS is produced.
Testosterone is produced.
Female sex ducts do not develop.
Male sex ducts fully develop.
DHT is made from testosterone.
Genitalia masculinize fully.

Figure 2.5

missing or did not function properly. These babies develop (1) internal female sex ducts in the absence of MIS, (2) no internal male sex ducts (because no testosterone was produced), and (3) female external genitalia (because no DHT was produced; figure 2.6).

Problems Responding to Testicular Hormones

All hormones have receptors that are found in parts of the body affected by those hormones. These receptors allow cells to respond to hormones. To respond to masculinizing hormones such as testosterone and DHT, there must be a sufficient number of functioning androgen receptors present. The term "androgens" refers to a group of masculinizing hormones that can be found in both men and women of which testosterone and DHT are the most potent. Without androgen receptors, the body cannot sense or respond to these masculinizing hormones.

Because development of the male sex ducts and external genitalia depend on the fetus's ability to respond to testosterone and DHT, babies who are 46,XY and lack functioning androgen receptors grow their reproductive anatomy in atypical ways. For example, if the receptors are partially broken, as happens in a condition called "partial androgen insensitivity syndrome" (PAIS; see figure 2.7), then the result is a person with (1) a 46,XY chromosomal complement, (2) testes (because *SRY* is present on the Y chromosome), (3) no internal female sex ducts (because the testes produce the hormone MIS), (4) partial development of the internal male sex ducts (because although the testes make testosterone, the male ducts

---

(*Opposite*) Figure 2.5. 46,XY DSD due to partial gonadal dysgenesis.
In partial gonadal dysgenesis (*top panel*), the testes are incompletely formed and do not produce enough Müllerian inhibiting substance (MIS) or testosterone at the right times during fetal development to result in male-typical reproductive structures. This hormonal environment may result in a situation where the internal reproductive structures of both boys (Wolffian) and girls (Müllerian) remain partially developed, and the external genitalia are ambiguous. Typical male differentiation is displayed in the bottom panel.

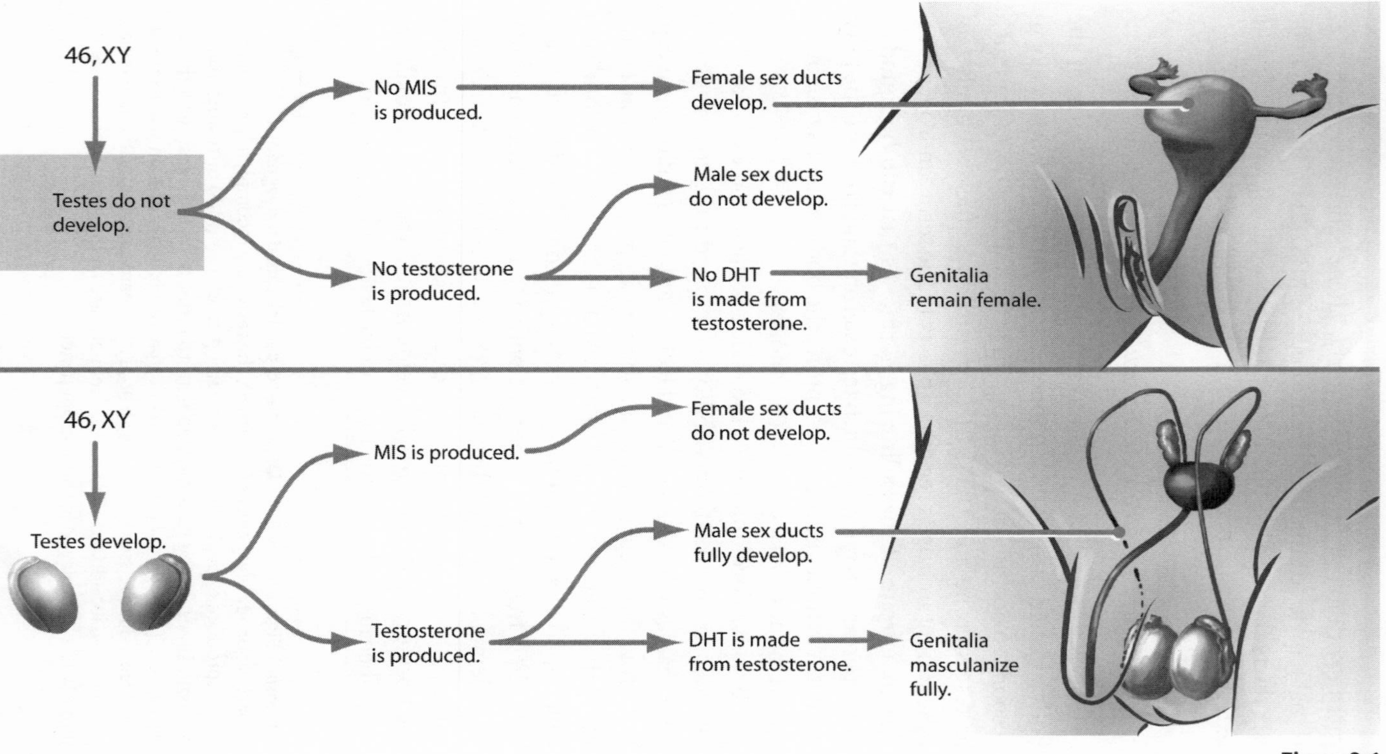
46, XY
Testes do not develop.
No MIS is produced.
No testosterone is produced.
Female sex ducts develop.
Male sex ducts do not develop.
No DHT is made from testosterone.
Genitalia remain female.
46, XY
Testes develop.
MIS is produced.
Testosterone is produced.
Female sex ducts do not develop.
Male sex ducts fully develop.
DHT is made from testosterone.
Genitalia masculanize fully.

Figure 2.6

cannot completely respond or develop in the presence of this hormone), and (5) ambiguous external genitalia (because the genital structures cannot completely respond to DHT).

Another condition with a similar cause is complete androgen insensitivity syndrome (CAIS). But this syndrome results in a very different experience for those affected. Androgen receptors are either completely missing or do not function at all in babies with CAIS. Although these babies are 46,XY and develop testes that produce male-typical amounts of testicular hormones, their bodies cannot sense the presence of testosterone and DHT and, as a result, babies with CAIS are born with (1) no internal female sex ducts (due to MIS action), (2) very limited internal male sex ducts (due to the inability to respond to testosterone), and (3) female external genitalia (due to the inability to respond to DHT; figure 2.8).

What Other Types of DSD Are There?

In addition to 46,XX DSD and 46,XY DSD, other types of DSD include sex chromosome DSD and ovotesticular DSD. Sex chromosome DSD refers to conditions with an atypical number of sex chromosomes, such as Klinefelter syndrome with two X chromosomes and one Y (47,XXY) and Turner syndrome with only one X chromosome and no Y (45,X). People with sex chromosome DSD are neither 46,XX nor 46,XY. Most affected individuals have problems with reproductive function and hormone production, but they are not born with ambiguous external genitalia or atypical internal sex ducts. Because of this, some people do not consider these conditions to be a type of DSD.

(*Opposite*) Figure 2.6. 46,XY DSD due to complete gonadal dysgenesis or Swyer syndrome.

In complete gonadal dysgenesis (*top panel*) the testes either never formed or were lost very early in fetal life. The lack of Müllerian inhibiting substance (MIS) and testosterone results in external genitals that are female typical and internal reproductive structures typical for a girl as well, except that ovaries are not present. The typical male differentiation is displayed in the bottom panel.

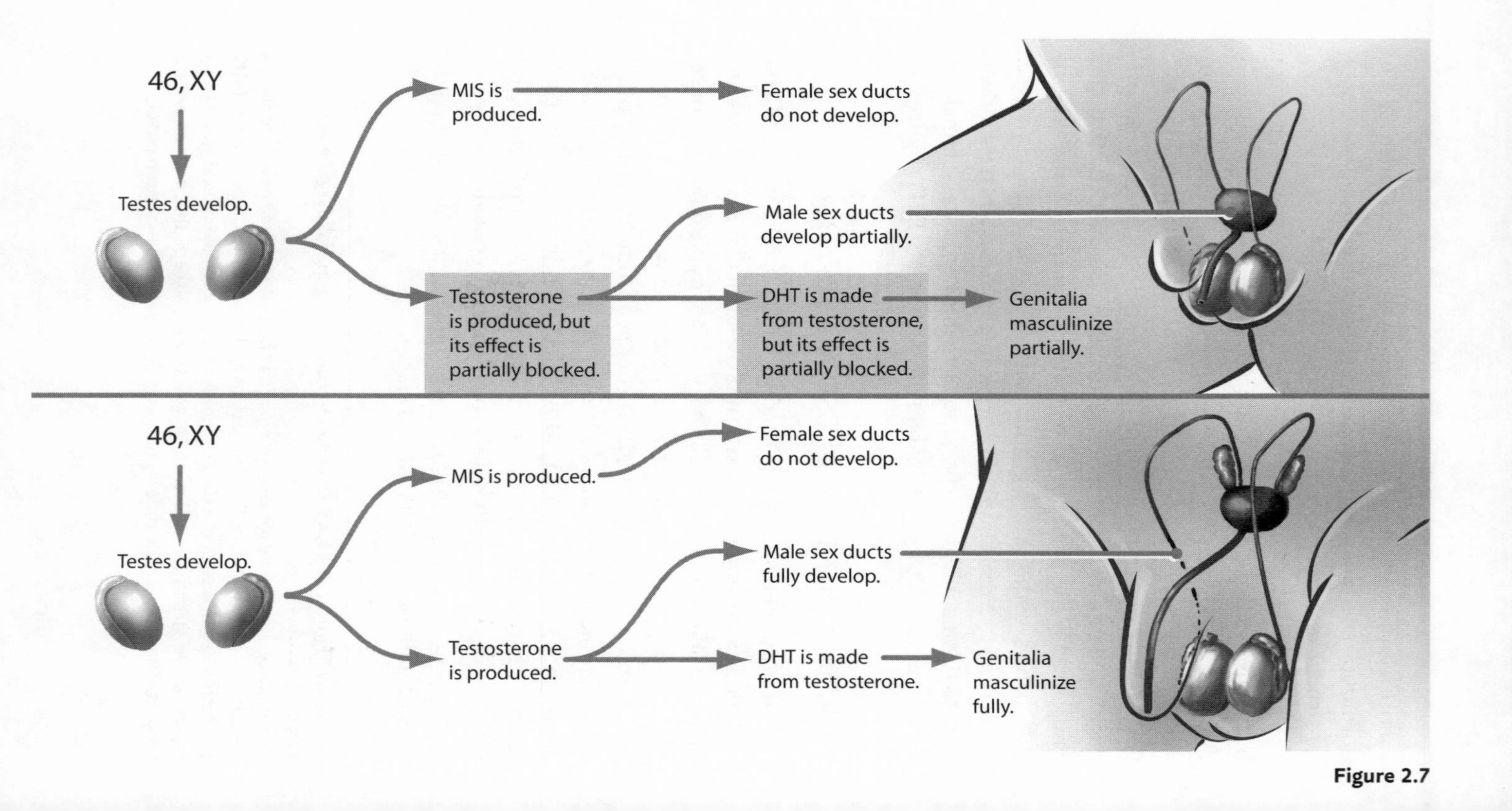
46, XY
Testes develop.
MIS is produced.
Female sex ducts do not develop.
Male sex ducts develop partially.
Testosterone is produced, but its effect is partially blocked.
DHT is made from testosterone, but its effect is partially blocked.
Genitalia masculinize partially.
46, XY
Testes develop.
MIS is produced.
Female sex ducts do not develop.
Male sex ducts fully develop.
Testosterone is produced.
DHT is made from testosterone.
Genitalia masculinize fully.

Figure 2.7

Ovotesticular DSD occurs when a child develops both ovaries and testes, instead of one or the other. Children with ovotesticular DSD can be 46,XX, 46,XY, or some other sex chromosome combination. Development of the internal and external genital structures is highly variable from one person to another person with ovotesticular DSD.

(*Opposite*) Figure 2.7. Sex differentiation in partial androgen insensitivity syndrome (PAIS).
In PAIS (*top panel*), testosterone is produced at levels that would ordinarily result in formation of complete male reproductive structures. The effect is blunted because the tissues cannot respond adequately due to a mutation in the androgen receptor gene. Therefore the external genitals appear ambiguous, but no internal female structures remain because Müllerian inhibiting substance (MIS) action is unimpeded. Testes are structurally normal in the womb and at birth. This differs from partial gonadal dysgenesis (Figure 2.5), in which some of the female internal reproductive structures are usually retained. The typical male differentiation is displayed in the bottom panel.

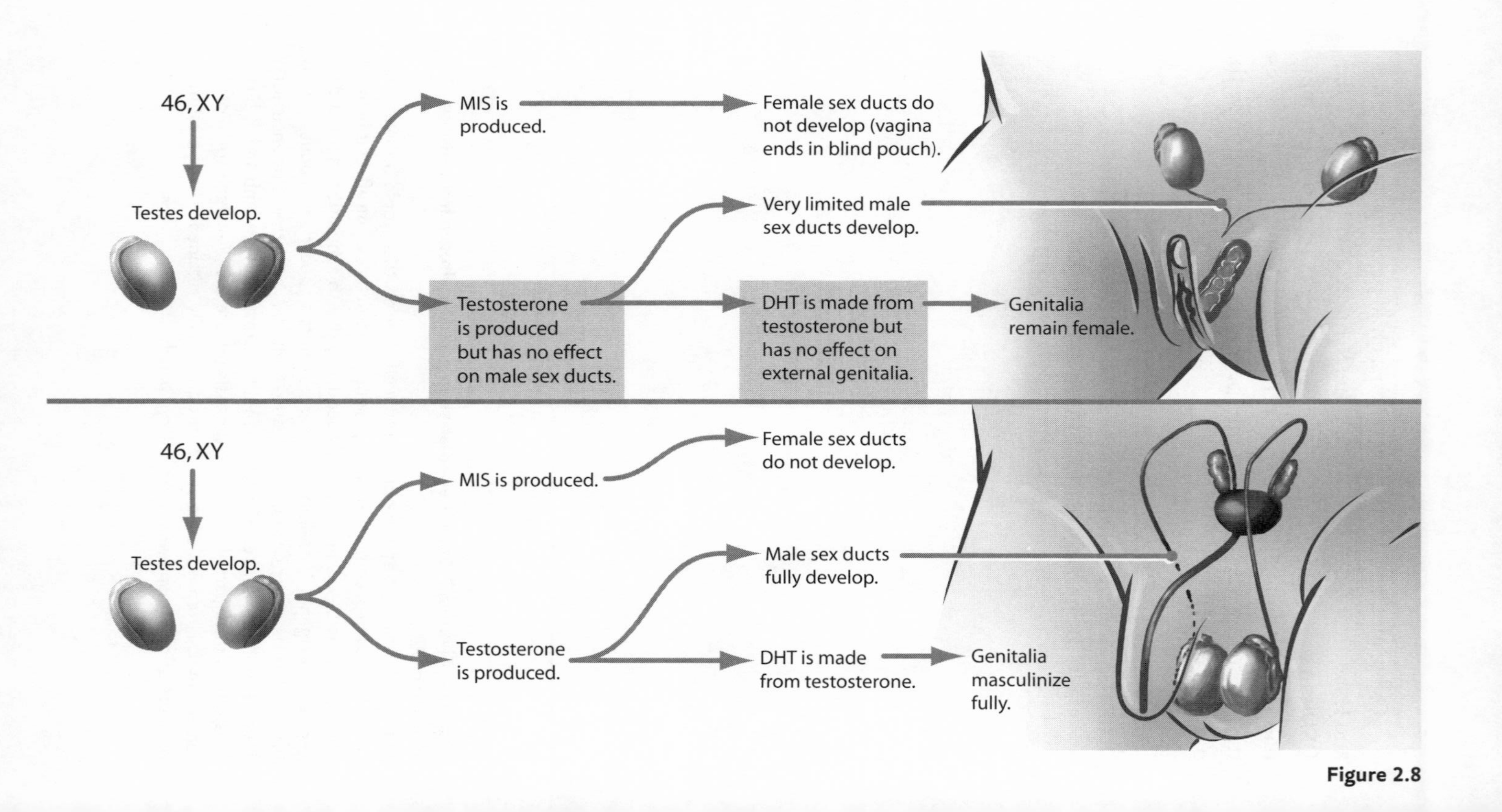
46, XY
Testes develop.
MIS is produced.
Female sex ducts do not develop (vagina ends in blind pouch).
Testosterone is produced but has no effect on male sex ducts.
Very limited male sex ducts develop.
DHT is made from testosterone but has no effect on external genitalia.
Genitalia remain female.
46, XY
Testes develop.
MIS is produced.
Female sex ducts do not develop.
Testosterone is produced.
Male sex ducts fully develop.
DHT is made from testosterone.
Genitalia masculinize fully.

Figure 2.8

• Chapter Summary •

DSD encompasses a wide array of medical conditions. We categorize DSD into three major groups—(1) 46,XX DSD, (2) 46,XY DSD, and (3) other types of DSD—to simplify how we think about these conditions. The specific testing needed and the medical approach recommended will depend on which category best fits your child's situation. Chapter 3 explains how your health care team determines which type of DSD affects your child, as well as which tests are needed to precisely define why the DSD occurred in the first place.

(*Opposite*) Figure 2.8. Sex differentiation in complete androgen insensitivity syndrome (CAIS).

In CAIS (*top panel*), testosterone is produced at levels typical or even high for a male fetus but the external genitalia remain female because the body is incapable of responding to testosterone. This happens when androgen receptors are missing or completely unable to function. Testes are structurally normal during fetal development and at birth, but in many cases they remain in the abdomen because there is no scrotum in which to descend. As in PAIS, no internal female structures remain because Müllerian inhibiting substance (MIS) action is unimpeded. Although the external appearance of complete gonadal dysgenesis (figure 2.6) and CAIS are similar, the internal anatomy is different. The typical male differentiation is displayed in the bottom panel.

• 3 •

How Will My Newborn Baby Be Evaluated?

Key Questions

How are different types of DSD identified?
What testing is used to establish a diagnosis?
How are these tests done?
What will these tests tell me about my baby's condition?

Many years ago, one of us was called to evaluate a baby born with ambiguous genitalia at a community hospital. The baby's pediatrician recounted that after examining the child, "at first I thought it was a boy, but then I thought it was a girl. In the end I stuck my neck out and said this was a boy." Testing later revealed that although the genitalia of this child was ambiguous, the recommended gender of rearing was female, because the infant was affected by 46,XX DSD due to CAH (see chapter 2 for a review of this diagnosis). What if this baby's parents had already assumed, based on the pediatrician's comment, that they had a son? When told about their daughter's CAH diagnosis, the parents said, "We could tell that the first doctor was uncertain about our baby's sex, and so we thought we would just wait until we had more information before deciding on a name."

This story illustrates the benefit of patience in assigning a sex to a newborn with DSD. Some people consider it a "medical emergency" when a newborn is suspected of having a DSD, but, while it is important to quickly identify life-threatening conditions that can be associated with DSD, incorrect assumptions about a newborn's sex or medical options can leave lasting, negative impressions on a family.

When evaluating a newborn with DSD, the first and most important goal is to identify and treat any life-threatening conditions that might be present. The second goal is to identify the category of DSD (as described in chapter 2) affecting the child. The third goal is to diagnose, when possible, the underlying cause of the DSD. The fourth and final goal is to define the specific reproductive anatomy of the baby, both internal and external. All of this information is then used to guide the treatment plan, including selecting the most appropriate gender of rearing. This information is obtained through a variety of tests, which are listed in table 3.1.

In this chapter we describe how doctors evaluate a newborn whom they think might have a DSD. We focus on the laboratory and imaging tests that are useful in checking your baby's health. We also consider how this information informs the treatment plan developed for your child.

Goal 1: Identifying Life-threatening Forms of DSD

Two kinds of life-threatening medical conditions occur in babies with DSD. The first involves deficiencies of the hormones produced by the adrenal glands, namely cortisol and aldosterone. As discussed in chapter 2, cortisol is a hormone that is necessary for the body to withstand physical stress. Aldosterone is a hormone that regulates salt balance. Babies who do not produce cortisol have problems with low blood sugar and show signs of weakness and poor feeding if not treated medically. The inability to produce aldosterone causes loss of salt in the urine, which can cause problems with the levels of sodium and potassium in the blood, poor weight gain, low blood pressure, and shock.

Although these hormone deficiencies are serious and poten-

Table 3.1. Useful Tests for Evaluating Newborns with DSD

Test	*Purpose*	*Procedure*	*Comment*
Karyotype	Assess chromosome number including the presence of X and Y	DNA from blood sample	Used for initial DSD categorization
FISH	Test for X and Y chromosomes and the *SRY* gene	DNA from blood sample	Rapid identification of sex chromosomes and testis determining factor
Adrenal hormones	Diagnose CAH	Blood sample	Standard testing for most forms of 46,XX DSD
Testicular hormones	Assess testis function 46,XY Diagnose 46,XY DSD	Blood sample	Standard testing for many forms of 46,XY DSD
Gene analysis	Diagnose specific mutations that cause DSD	DNA from blood sample	Can help determine risk for other family members or future pregnancies
HCG stimulation	Assess testis function	Measure testosterone and DHT production after hCG injections	Standard testing for many forms of 46,XY DSD
Pelvic ultrasound	Locate Müllerian structures and gonads	Ultrasound takes a picture of internal reproductive structures	Dependent on expert interpretation
Vaginogram	Define lower reproductive tract anatomy	Special x-ray using a dye in the lower reproductive tract	Clarifies ultrasound results
Vaginoscopy/cystoscopy	Define lower reproductive tract anatomy	Direct visualization procedure under general anesthesia	Defines anatomy of the bladder and urogenital sinus
Laparoscopy	Define internal anatomy, gonad biopsy when necessary	Minimally invasive surgical procedure under anesthesia	Helpful in diagnosing dysgenetic testes or ovotesticular DSD

Note: DSD = disorder of sex development; CAH = congenital adrenal hyperplasia; hCG = human chorionic gonadotropin. The terms 46,XX and 46,XY refer to the typical number of chromosomes (46) and either female (XX) or male (XY) chromosomes. Müllerian structures refer to early versions of female internal genitalia that are found in all fetuses but generally disappear at a certain stage in male fetuses.

tially life-threatening, their diagnosis is usually straightforward and their treatment is effective. The type of DSD category that affects your child, coupled with the appearance of your baby's internal and external reproductive anatomy, will alert your child's doctor to whether your child needs testing for cortisol and aldosterone deficiencies. We will talk more about how these tests are done in the following sections.

The second cause of life-threatening conditions in newborns with DSD is problems with organ development. Formation of the kidneys, gastrointestinal tract, and cardiovascular system may be incomplete in some newborns with DSD. Most often physical signs point to the need for concern. If your baby appears healthy in all ways except for the development of his or her reproductive structures, it is unlikely that there are problems with other major organ systems. Again, the category of your child's DSD, coupled with the appearance of his or her reproductive structures, will allow your child's doctor to determine if the health of your baby's kidneys, gastrointestinal tract, or cardiovascular system needs to be evaluated.

Goal 2: Finding out Which Category of DSD Your Child Has

The second goal of a medical evaluation is to determine whether your child is affected by 46,XX DSD, 46,XY DSD, or another form of DSD. As you might expect, your child's doctor needs to gather information about your baby's sex chromosomes to answer this question. There are two ways to do this. The first is to perform a count of the chromosomes found in cells of any tissue, which is called a "standard karyotype." Nearly every cell in our bodies has the same number (46) of chromosomes, so it usually does not matter which cells are used for karyotype testing. Typically, white blood cells are used because these are easy to obtain. A small blood sample that contains white cells is collected and then examined. If the karyotype is 46,XX, then there are 46 chromosomes in total (the typical number for humans) including two X chromosomes. Alternatively, if the baby's karyotype is 46,XY, then there are 46 chromosomes in total including an X and a Y chromosome.

Another test commonly performed, often in conjunction with a standard karyotype, is a special test called "fluorescence in situ hybridization," or FISH. It can be used to rapidly determine the presence or absence of certain DNA sequences in a chromosome. In evaluating DSD, the presence of the X or Y chromosomes overall or the *SRY* gene specifically are tested for. Remember that this gene, which is usually present on the Y chromosome, determines whether testes form or not. (We reviewed this in the section on gonadal development in chapter 1.) If *SRY* is present, then the entire Y chromosome is usually present as well. Some babies who have a 46,XX karyotype do have the *SRY* gene on one of their X chromosomes or on one of their other chromosomes, and the presence of that gene would be missed by standard karyotype testing alone.

Sometimes parents are told their baby's karyotype before birth as a result of prenatal testing, such as when a mother has a biopsy of the placenta or a sample of her amniotic cells. When DSD is suspected due to ambiguous genitalia at birth, or when the prenatal test results do not match the anatomical sex of the baby at birth, a repeat karyotype may be needed. Your child's doctor will let you know if it is necessary to repeat any tests that were performed before your baby was born.

DSD categorization is generally straightforward. If your child's karyotype is 46,XX, then the correct category is 46,XX DSD; if your child's karyotype is 46,XY, then your child is affected by some type of 46,XY DSD. However, not all forms of DSD are covered by these two general categories. The "other" category of DSD includes individuals who have an atypical chromosome number. For example, some people with DSD have some cells that are 45,X (that is, those cells are missing one sex chromosome) and other cells that are 46,XY. For these people their combination of sex chromosomes differs from cell to cell, resulting in a condition called "mosaicism." Ovotesticular DSD (see chapter 2) affects people with a 46,XX karyotype, a 46,XY karyotype, or some other combination of sex chromosomes. Ovotesticular DSD occurs when both ovaries and testes develop in a single individual. Because sex chromosomes vary among individuals with ovotesticular DSD, this condition is not usually diagnosed by a karyotype; instead, other laboratory or imaging studies are used to make this determination.

Goal 3: Finding out What Caused Your Child's DSD

Congenital Adrenal Hyperplasia and 46,XX DSD

As noted previously, CAH is by far the most common cause of 46,XX DSD. Affected newborns show variable degrees of masculinization of their external genitalia including phallic enlargement and labial fusion to form what looks like an underdeveloped penis and scrotum. However, these children possess ovaries, a uterus, and fallopian tubes. This discrepancy occurs because excess testosterone production by the adrenal glands, which is converted to DHT in the body, masculinizes the external genitalia. These children have ovaries because their two X chromosomes do not include the *SRY* gene. Their internal female structures form normally because no testes were present to produce MIS. Recall that a fetus will have both female (Müllerian) and male (Wolffian) ducts at some point in development. MIS typically causes the female structures to disappear, leaving the male ones to develop in boys.

The diagnosis of CAH is made by a blood test that measures levels of adrenal hormones. Specifically, in CAH, blood levels of the hormone 17-hydroxyprogesterone (17-OHP) are elevated. When performed correctly, testing for levels of 17-OHP in the blood confirms the diagnosis of CAH 95 percent of the time. The remaining individuals who have CAH are unable to produce the enzyme 11β-hydroxylase. Testing for 11β-hydroxylase deficiency is similar to that for diagnosing 21-hydroxylase deficiency; levels of 11-deoxycortisol in the blood are measured to diagnose this rarer form of CAH.

For newborns with CAH, the diagnosis is almost always made by a single blood test. On rare occasions, additional testing may be needed. These additional tests generally fall into two categories. First are tests in which hormones are given to the infant to stimulate the adrenal glands to produce cortisol and aldosterone. These stimulation tests are designed to uncover adrenal gland abnormalities that are not apparent with a single blood test. Figure 2.3 in chapter 2 shows the connection between the adrenocorticotrophic hormone (ACTH) and the masculinizing hormone DHT. ACTH primarily regulates secretion of cortisol, which is impaired in all forms of CAH. The ACTH test is sometimes needed to pinpoint the biochemical step that is affected (hence the type of CAH) or to magnify the effects of a mild form and thereby establish the diagnosis. Thus, ACTH stimulation tests are typically used in older children who have mild forms of CAH that do not include ambiguous genitalia at birth, but they are sometimes needed for infants with rare forms of CAH.

Other tests that may be employed for diagnosing CAH include examining your baby's genes for mutations that cause CAH. This type of testing is done by getting DNA from a blood sample and sending it to a laboratory for analysis. When genetic testing is used, doctors interpreting the tests need to be expert in doing so; if questions about the interpretations arise, genetic specialists and counselors can help.

SRY *Translocation and 46,XX DSD*

A form of 46,XX DSD that is not due to CAH occurs in individuals with an *SRY* translocation. Their karyotype is 46,XX, but the *SRY* gene (normally present on the Y chromosome) has been inserted into one of their other chromosomes. Because *SRY* is present, testes develop (although incompletely for some people), resulting in masculinized genitalia in a genetic female. The diagnosis of *SRY* translocation is made when a child with a 46,XX karyotype is born with ambiguous genitalia but in whom no form of

CAH is identified. A FISH test that detects the presence of the *SRY* gene on any chromosome can confirm this diagnosis. Adrenal gland function is normal in this type of DSD.

Problems with Testicular Hormone Production and 46,XY DSD

Diagnosing 46,XY DSD is more challenging than diagnosing 46,XX DSD, because the potential causes of 46,XY DSD are more varied. A specific diagnosis is reached in only half of all newborns with 46,XY DSD despite extensive laboratory testing. Even when a diagnosis is not reached, your medical team can work with you to develop a successful treatment plan for your baby. Explanations of various treatment plans are offered in chapter 5.

In newborns with a 46,XY karyotype, the main source of testosterone is the testes. If testicular production of testosterone is insufficient during critical periods of prenatal development (when the genitalia are forming), then 46,XY DSD results. Testosterone production may be low because the testosterone-producing (Leydig) cells are absent in the developing testes or because the Leydig cells are present but lack the enzymes needed to produce testosterone. In newborns with a 46,XY karyotype who are unable to produce normal amounts of testosterone, the testicles may be normal in size and may also produce male-typical levels of the hormone MIS. For these children, the external genitalia will be underdeveloped and will appear ambiguous or more typical of a female but no internal Müllerian (female) organs will be present. In contrast, in children with a 46,XY karyotype who experience problems with formation of the entire testis (the Leydig cells as well as other cell types), both testosterone and MIS production may be insufficient to support male-typical reproductive development. In these newborns, internal Müllerian structures are sometimes present.

A diagnosis of insufficient testicular hormone production in newborns with 46,XY DSD is reached through a combination of anatomical features observed during a genital exam (ambiguous or female-typical genitalia) and blood test results. Measuring testosterone and MIS can identify whether the problem is limited to the Leydig cells or whether the child's testicular dysfunction is more extensive. Imaging tests such as pelvic ultrasounds reveal the presence or absence of internal Müllerian structures.

Though a simple, single blood sample may reveal a diagnosis of insufficient testicular hormone production, more complex testing is usually needed, because the production of testicular hormones is highly variable in young babies. Usually, a newborn's testes produce significant amounts of testosterone during the first months of life and then stop producing this hormone at around 4 months. Sometimes physicians will take blood samples from babies at 2 or 3 months to assess this early peak in testicular hormone production. If a baby is being evaluated for 46,XY DSD after the early peak has passed, then specific stimulation tests may be used to determine whether the testes can produce testosterone and MIS. One way to do this is to give the baby a hormone called hCG (human chorionic gonadotrophin), administered in a series of intramuscular injections, to stimulate testosterone production. Following these injections, a blood sample is taken from the child to measure his or her ability to produce testosterone, DHT, and sometimes other hormones.

Although for many children with 46,XY DSD the only problem is their impaired ability to make testosterone from the Leydig cells, for others additional hormone deficiencies can occur. For a child with multiple hormone deficiencies, diagnoses are usually made with a single blood sample that measures levels of several hormones. Occasionally, a stimulation test may be used to help determine when multiple hormone deficiencies exist in a baby with 46,XY DSD.

Problems with Testicular Hormone Action and 46,XY DSD

Some babies with 46,XY DSD produce normal amounts of testicular hormones, but the cells in their bodies are unable to respond to these hormones. These babies are also born with external genitalia that may appear ambiguous or female typical. Although the testes may be located in the abdomen rather than in the scrotum, their hormone production can be male typical. Newborns who have normal production of MIS will not have a uterus or fallopian tubes. For 46,XY babies born with female external genitalia who produce normal levels of testosterone and DHT, and in whom the internal Müllerian structures are absent, the cause of DSD may be complete androgen insensitivity syndrome (CAIS). The only definitive test for diagnosing androgen insensitivity syndrome is a genetic study that examines androgen receptor gene structure. This study can be done by taking DNA from a blood sample and sending it to a specialized lab for analysis. Genetic tests can also be helpful in diagnosing partial androgen insensitivity syndrome (PAIS) that results in ambiguous genitalia in newborns with a 46,XY karyotype.

Sometimes 46,XY DSD is associated with physical abnormalities such as underdevelopment of major organ systems or overall stunted growth of the entire baby while in the womb. These indicate a syndrome—a group of clinical features that are commonly found together—of 46,XY DSD and are thought to be relatively rare. When syndromic forms of 46,XY DSD are suspected, parents and doctors can consult with a medical genetics specialist who can provide information about what to expect for affected children as they grow, as well as about the chance of recurrence in future pregnancies.

Goal 4: Understanding Your Child's Anatomy

Knowing a specific diagnosis for your child goes a long way in shaping his or her treatment plan, including which gender of rearing is best and what genital surgery, if any, should be performed. Parents can make the best treatment decisions for their child in consultation with their child's physicians when they have a complete understanding of their child's reproductive anatomy and diagnosis. The degree of overmasculinization or undermasculinization of reproductive structures varies from child to child, even among affected children within the same family. For parents of more than one child with DSD, especially, this is good information to know. Here we explain how physicians precisely define reproductive anatomy in newborns affected by DSD.

External Genitalia: Description and Characterization

A detailed examination of the external genitalia is performed to measure the length and width of your child's phallus, the quality of the erectile tissue within the phallus (also called corpora cavernosa, or corporal bodies), the presence or absence of descended testes, and the location of the urethral meatus (where your baby's urine exits the body). Such an examination is highly important for predicting responses to future medical therapy as well as understanding what to expect if parents choose to proceed with genital surgery. For children who have female-typical genitalia, the labia and clitoris will be examined.

Examination of Internal Reproductive Structures

In addition to accurately defining the anatomy of the external genitalia, several other pieces of information may be needed for planning your child's medical treatment, including the following: *Where are the gonads located and are they healthy? Are Müllerian structures (internal female sex organs) present and are they completely formed? Are Wolffian structures (internal male sex organs) present and are they completely formed? Does my baby have a urogenital sinus? If so, is the urogenital sinus big? Where is the urogenital sinus located?*

A "urogenital sinus" develops when the urinary tract and vagina merge together before exiting the body. A urogenital sinus is sometimes present in newborns with ambiguous genitalia. The relationship between a baby's urinary outflow and development and position of the vagina determines what will be required for either masculinizing or feminizing surgery, if parents opt for that approach. The size and location of the urogenital sinus can be determined by multiple kinds of imaging studies or direct visualization during surgical procedures. Each procedure has specific advantages and limitations and is described below.

PELVIC ULTRASONOGRAPHY

This imaging test can be performed on a baby at any age and is similar to the ultrasounds a woman receives during pregnancy. Pelvic ultrasonography identifies the presence and degree of development of Müllerian structures. This test is both simple and safe and uses an ultrasound probe that is touched to the baby's lower abdomen. The advantages of pelvic ultrasonography are its ease of operation and the quick and rapid identification of internal anatomy. It can also identify whether gonads are ovaries, testes, or ovotestes. Pelvic ultrasonography is less well-suited for examining lower reproductive anatomy such as the vagina or determining the structure of the urogenital sinus. The key to getting useful information from a pelvic ultrasound is to have this test performed and interpreted by a professional who is experienced in the evaluation of infants. When the test is performed by inexperienced technicians, important findings are easily missed.

MAGNETIC RESONANCE IMAGING (MRI)

This form of imaging test provides a more detailed examination of the internal reproductive structures than is provided by an ultrasound. It can also examine other organs within the baby's abdomen. MRIs give much of the same information that's obtained with pelvic ultrasound, but they can better identify any problems that may exist. Similarly to pelvic ultrasounds, MRIs are not good at defining lower reproductive anatomy such as a urogenital sinus.

To have an MRI, a baby is placed in a large scanning device and must remain relatively still for a few minutes so that the MRI machine can obtain a good image. Like ultrasounds, MRIs are safe and painless, but the machine can be noisy and can startle the child. MRIs require a person to remain still. The likelihood that a baby will move during the test means that sedation is required to obtain optimal MRI results.

CYSTOGRAMS AND VAGINOGRAMS

These imaging tests are x-ray studies that use a small amount of dye infused into the lower reproductive or urinary tract. These tests are better than ultrasound or MRI at defining lower reproductive structures. Cystograms and vaginograms can identify the bladder, Müllerian structures, and the urogenital sinus when these exist. These tests are safe despite the small amount of radiation exposure from the x-rays.

CYSTOSCOPY AND VAGINOSCOPY

For some babies there is a need for direct visualization of the lower urinary tract. Tests called cystoscopy (looking into the bladder) and vaginoscopy (looking into the vagina or urogenital sinus) are used to better define the anatomy of the lower reproductive tract. With these imaging techniques, doctors can tell whether a vagina is present, where it is located, and whether there is a cervix present at the end of the vagina.

For these procedures, infants are given general anesthesia, and a very small flexible device is then inserted into the vagina, urogenital sinus, or urethra. The physician will examine the anatomy of these structures and take pictures of important features. These procedures are relatively quick and generally harmless, but they do involve the risk of general anesthesia. They only image the lower parts of a child's reproductive anatomy; they cannot directly examine gonads or the upper portions of the Müllerian ducts. These procedures are usually performed by a pediatric urologist or a similarly trained surgeon.

LAPAROSCOPY

This surgical procedure is performed when direct visualization of the gonads or other internal reproductive structures, or a biopsy of these structures, is necessary for making a diagnosis or developing a treatment plan for a child with DSD. For laparoscopy the child is under general anesthesia. Small incisions are made through the skin of the lower abdomen, and then a scope is passed through a small incision to allow the surgeon to directly visualize the internal structures. Biopsies are taken of the gonads (a biopsy involves cutting and collecting a small sample of tissue). After examination of the biopsies in a laboratory, it can be determined whether the gonads are testes or a mixture of testes and ovaries (ovotesticular DSD). Biopsy results can also reveal whether the gonads are healthy or are at risk for developing tumors. Though uncommon, biopsy can result in unintended damage to or loss of the gonad.

The Next Step

Sometimes the most relevant medical information regarding your child's DSD can be gathered in only a few days, and his or her medical plan can be laid out soon after birth. For other children, more extensive, time-consuming testing may be required. Tests are completed within the first weeks of life for most newborns. Once testing has been completed, the next step is to discuss the results with your child's health care team and then define a treatment plan, including (1) a gender of rearing, (2) medical interventions (if any), and (3) genital surgery (if any).

Chapter 4 reviews how decisions are made regarding gender assignment for newborns with DSD. Chapter 5 describes how parents and doctors develop medical treatment plans for newborns with DSD, as well as what to expect for your son's or daughter's long-term medical care. We also begin to weigh the pros and cons of medical and surgical treatment options, such as the timing of removal of testes in cases in which they are at risk for developing tumors and the appropriate age for surgery to alter the cosmetic appearance of ambiguous external genitalia.

• *Chapter Summary* •

When a baby is born with ambiguous genitalia, a series of tests are performed to establish the best treatment plan for that child. The prompt initiation of a meaningful evaluation is important, and physicians should strive to collect relevant information about a newborn's DSD in a reasonable time frame. Nonetheless, it is important to allow the laboratory testing and imaging studies to follow a logical course and not to be hasty with decisions or draw conclusions that are incomplete or incorrect. Such haste will only cause undue stress for the family and complicate the child's medical management.

Categorizing the type of DSD (46,XX, 46,XY, or other) is usually straightforward. Reaching a specific diagnosis within the general categories of DSD is more involved. Even when a specific diagnosis cannot be determined, information gathered from tests may reveal an optimal gender assignment and medical and surgical treatment plans. Your child's health care team should explain what tests your child needs and why and should keep you informed of the results so that you can make the best possible decisions for your baby. If you do not feel that you are being given the information you need, ask your child's physicians. Generally there is at least one person on the health care team who is good at interacting with parents, and this person will be the one you turn to most often when you need information.

• 4 •

Gender Development in DSD

Key Questions

What is gender?
What is known about long-term gender development in people with DSD?

When a baby is born with DSD, many parents ask, "Is my baby a boy or a girl?" Unfortunately, some parents receive conflicting answers to this question. Naturally, they become frustrated and confused when they get contradictory advice from health care professionals about the best gender of rearing for their child.

This chapter explains what gender is and describes the long-term development of gender in individuals who grew up with DSD. While we cannot predict future gender identity with complete certainty for any newborn (affected by DSD or not), research has revealed patterns of behavioral development that guide treatment plans for newborns with specific types of DSD. Overall, the chapter will clarify how this information influences recommendations for gender assignment in affected newborns.

What Is Gender?

The words "gender" and "sex" are often used interchangeably, but the two words have different meanings. While sex refers to the biological characteristics (chromosomes, gonads, hormones) that distinguish boys from girls, gender refers to the behaviors that distinguish the sexes. Girls and boys differ in many ways according to their gender. First, girls usually identify themselves as female, while boys usually see themselves as male. The identification with one sex over the other is called "gender identity." One of the most important goals in developing a treatment plan for newborns with DSD is to have a child develop a gender identity that matches their upbringing. *Note: Throughout this chapter, recommendations for gender assignment are meant for newborns with DSD only. Older children who have already established a gender identity should not be subjected to male or female reassignment unless the child requests such a change.*

A second component of gender is the public expression of sex-typed behavior, referred to as "gender role." For example, a girl may prefer hunting or sports to playing with dolls and a boy may be more interested in fashion design than in playing sports. For these children, their gender identity is female and male, respectively. But their gender role may be considered atypical (but not incorrect or unhealthy).

The third and final aspect of gender is "sexual orientation." Most people are sexually attracted to members of the opposite sex and are thus classified as heterosexual. A significant number of people are sexually attracted to members of the same sex and are referred to as homosexual. Some people are attracted to both sexes (bisexual) while others experience no sexual attraction at all to other people (asexual). While gender identity is a significant factor in deciding on a gender assignment for newborns with DSD, neither gender role nor sexual orientation is usually considered when deciding on a gender assignment for newborns with DSD. Gender role and sexual orientation are not taken into account because they cannot be determined in infancy. Also, even if these aspects of behavior could be determined in young children, society is becoming less rigid in its expectations of what hobbies or interests are appropriate for girls and boys and a diversity of sexual orientation is also increasingly being accepted by society.

We know a lot about how male and female *sex* develops. In the previous chapters we learned how genes like *SRY* and hormones like testosterone orchestrate the complex development of a human baby into a fully formed female or male. If we had the same level of understanding about gender identity, then we would have tests to correctly identify gender early on, and we would know the age when gender identity becomes established. Unfortunately, we know little about the mechanisms involved in the development of gender identity. Is gender identity determined by specific genes or by exposure of the brain to sex hormones or is it something that is learned from the way a child is reared during formative years? At what age can we be comfortable that a child born with DSD is being raised in the appropriate gender? It is probable that genes, hormones, and environment all combine to determine a child's gender identity, but it is not yet known which of these variables dominate in children with DSD.

Despite these gaps in our understanding, many things that we do know can give you comfort as you decide on the gender of rearing for your baby. First, for many forms of DSD there are data that indicate that there will be a high probability that gender identity will match rearing. Second, for most people with DSD, gender identity is evident within the first few years of life. Third, for DSD conditions where the future gender identity is less predictable, a plan that optimizes outcome can be developed. Finally, in the unlikely event that a person with DSD will desire a change in gender, this can be managed. (We discuss gender change in more detail in chapter 9.)

Gender Development in People with DSD

21-Hydroxylase Deficiency

As mentioned earlier, research has revealed patterns of behavioral development that guide treatment plans for newborns with specific types of DSD. For example, in congenital adrenal hyperplasia due to 21-hydroxylase deficiency, which is the most common form of 46,XX DSD, female gender identity develops in the vast majority (95%) of babies who are reared as girls. This outcome, coupled with the potential for successful future pregnancies once the child reaches womanhood, is the basis for recommending female gender for these children despite their masculinized external genitalia. That said, some medical professionals consider male rearing in genetic females with severely masculinized genitalia due to CAH.

While gender role and sexual orientation are not usually considered when deciding on a gender assignment for newborn girls with CAH, it is important to educate parents about behaviors that their daughters are likely to exhibit as they grow up. First, these girls have a higher than average interest in sports and are often excellent athletes. As they develop further into adulthood, women with CAH often pursue male-dominated careers such as auto mechanics. We encourage parents to support their daughters' interests in sports and physical activity. Participating in athletics is an important part of maintaining health and building self-esteem, and there is no reason to discourage such behavior. Furthermore, interest in male-dominated careers can often lead to good earning potential and career advancement for women. These are just some examples of how gender role can be atypical in girls and women with CAH but not incorrect or unhealthy.

In the area of sexual orientation, the majority of women with CAH are heterosexual. However, women with CAH are more likely to report a bisexual or homosexual orientation than unaffected women. About 20% of women with CAH are sexually attracted to other women. (Note that most homosexual women do not have CAH.) It is unknown at this time the extent to which hormone status prior to or during treatment influences rates of heterosexuality or homosexuality in women with CAH. Chapter 5 discusses medical and surgical treatments commonly recommended for girls and women with CAH.

11β-Hydroxylase Deficiency or Other Causes

Less is known about gender development in people with 46,XX DSD resulting from 11β-hydroxylase deficiency or other causes than is known about gender development in people with 46,XX DSD resulting from 21-hydroxylase deficiency. Using the same approach in 11β-hydroxylase deficiency as we would for 21-hydroxylase deficiency makes sense because the conditions are very similar in their sex hormone profile, internal and external genital features, medical treatment, and potential for future fertility. So, female gender is recommended for newborns with 46,XX DSD due to 11β-hydroxylase deficiency.

For babies with 46,XX DSD resulting from problems with placental function or maternal tumors that expose the fetus to androgens prior to birth, female assignment is also recommended because ovaries and Müllerian ducts are present and allow these children to carry successful pregnancies when they grow up.

Problems with Testicular Hormone Production

For newborns *completely* unable to produce the testicular hormones testosterone and DHT (and sometimes MIS), female gender assignment is usually recommended despite the presence of a Y chromosome. An example of such a condition is Swyer syndrome (also known as "complete gonadal dysgenesis"; see figure 2.6). Newborns with Swyer syndrome have fully formed female internal sex ducts and external genitalia, even though they have a 46,XY chromosomal makeup. The testes in women with Swyer syndrome never formed properly. With hormone replacement at puberty, these children grow breasts and menstruate. Women with this condition successfully carry pregnancies after receiving donated, fertilized eggs.

When raised as girls, children with Swyer syndrome develop a female gender identity. Girls and women with 46,XY DSD due to complete gonadal dysgenesis are interested in pursuits that are typical among women and often report a female heterosexual orientation. If your baby is completely unable to produce testosterone and DHT for any number of reasons and your newborn has female external genitalia, then it is likely that female gender assignment will be recommended.

Newborns with XY sex chromosomes who produce testicular hormones but not enough of them for complete masculinization may be reared male or female. These children are born with ambiguous external genitalia. Chapter 3 explains how a detailed examination of the internal reproductive structures and external genitalia is conducted. Results from such examinations often influence recommendations for male or female assignment.

While many children reared male or female accept their gender assignment, dissatisfaction with *either* sex of rearing occurs most often in people with 46,XY DSD who were born with ambiguous genitalia. Because the likelihood of rejecting a gender assignment is greater among people with 46,XY DSD and ambiguous genitalia at birth, the medical community is increasingly recommending male sex assignment for those newborns. This is in part because the surgical treatments associated with being raised as a female (discussed in chapter 5) cannot be reversed if a child or adult develops a male gender identity despite having had a female upbringing.

Two conditions that fall under the general category 46,XY DSD resulting from problems with testicular hormone production require special mention because of the high likelihood that affected individuals will develop a male gender identity even though their genitals are very feminine in appearance at birth. These are 5α-reductase type 2 (5α-RD-2) and 17β-hydroxysteroid dehydrogenase-3 (17β-HSD-3) deficiencies. For both conditions, virilization at the age of puberty can be expected and for 5α-RD-2 deficiency specifically, fertility is possible with male (but not female) rearing. Therefore, male assignment may be recommended for children with either of these conditions, even with very undermasculinized genitals.

Problems Responding to Testicular Hormones

For newborns with complete androgen insensitivity syndrome (CAIS), that is, those who are *completely* unable to respond to testosterone and DHT, female gender assignment is recommended despite the presence of a Y chromosome and testes. Girls and women with CAIS develop a female gender identity, female-typical hobbies and interests, and often report a heterosexual orientation. In contrast, newborns with *partial* androgen insensitivity syndrome (PAIS) who have a blunted response to testosterone and DHT may be raised female or male. Recommendation for male versus female rearing in newborns with PAIS is influenced by the degree of insensitivity the child shows toward testosterone and DHT. A thorough examination of the genitalia can be helpful in making this assessment. As they do with 46,XY DSD due to problems with testicular hormone production, doctors are increasingly recommending male gender assignment for newborns with PAIS. Again, this is because surgery performed on children reared as female cannot be reversed if the child later identifies as male.

45,X/46,XY DSD, 46,XX/46,XY DSD, and Ovotesticular DSD

Newborns affected by 45,X/46,XY DSD or 46,XX/46,XY DSD have historically been raised male or female, depending on the degree of undermasculinization of the external genitalia at birth. When people in this group initiate gender reassignment, it is typically in the direction from female to male. In contrast, newborns with ovotesticular DSD are usually raised female because of the belief that doing so will optimize fertility potential for people with this condition. At the present time, we have limited knowledge of long-term gender development in people with any of these types of DSD, which are categorized as "other." As with previously discussed categories of DSD, feminizing surgery is avoided if male gender identity development is likely.

Sex Chromosome DSD

Gender assignment is not an issue for newborns affected by Klinefelter or Turner syndrome, both examples of sex chromosome DSD (see chapter 2). This is because the external genitalia of newborns with Klinefelter syndrome are male with no atypical features. Similarly, the external genitalia for newborns with Turner syndrome are female with no atypical features. Boys and men with Klinefelter syndrome develop a male gender identity, and girls and women with Turner syndrome develop a female gender identity. Furthermore, assisted reproductive technologies are increasingly resulting in fertility for men with Klinefelter syndrome and women with Turner syndrome.

• *Chapter Summary* •

When a baby is born with DSD, assigning a particular gender for that individual can be stressful. Knowing how adults who grew up with DSD developed long-term gender identity is useful for doctors when they recommend male or female assignment for infants. Chapter 3 discussed the importance of knowing what category of DSD affects your child. This knowledge will help you and your child's doctors make the most appropriate decision regarding gender assignment.

In general, babies with 46,XX DSD are reared female because the vast majority of these children develop a female gender identity. Babies with 46,XY DSD due to (1) a complete inability to make testosterone and DHT or (2) CAIS are also reared as girls because female gender identity is most likely for people with these conditions. Babies with 46,XY DSD due to (1) a partial inability to produce testicular hormones or (2) PAIS can be raised female or male, depending on the degree of masculinization of the genitalia. For newborns in either of these groups, parents should understand that dissatisfaction with sex of rearing occurs in some people, whether raised male or female. Being aware of this potential for dissatisfaction may influence later medical and surgical recommendations for the child. Finally, male assignment is recommended for newborns with 46,XY DSD due to 5α-RD-2 and 17β-HSD-3 deficiencies because of the high likelihood of their developing a male gender identity.

Once you and your child's doctors reach an agreement on the most appropriate gender of rearing for your child with DSD, the next step is to develop a long-term treatment plan that may involve surgery and daily medication. Chapter 5 describes common medical and surgical treatments recommended for infants and children with DSD and reviews the pros and cons associated with each one.

· 5 ·

Understanding and Weighing the Treatment Options

Key Questions

What medical treatments are available for infants and children with DSD?
What surgical treatments are available for infants and children with DSD?
What are the pros and cons associated with these treatments?

Understanding DSD is helpful in reducing the anxiety that surrounds the diagnosis and in paving the way for making informed decisions about medical and surgical treatment. These decisions can be difficult for parents. In this chapter, we explain the current treatment options available for infants and children with DSD and the benefits and drawbacks that can be associated with each. We believe this information will give you a better grasp of the medical choices you will make as a parent. We encourage you to use this chapter as an educational guide rather than as a prescription to rigidly follow. You know your child best. Together with your child's health care team, you will be able to develop an optimal treatment plan for your son or daughter.

Ideally, any treatment plan will be explained fully to you, including the advantages and disadvantages of proceeding with care versus not proceeding. You should be provided with enough information and time to make informed decisions for your child, including time to get a second opinion if you choose. Getting a second opinion is commonly done, and your child's health care team will almost certainly—and should—welcome a second opinion. (Chapter 8 explains how to go about pursuing this option.) When a family finds it difficult to locate an experienced team to help their child, patient advocate groups can provide contact information to medical centers that specialize in DSD treatment. (Information about such groups is provided in chapter 9.)

Medical Treatment: Pros and Cons

Parents' choices about medical treatment depend greatly on the type of DSD that affects their child as well as their child's gender of rearing. Generally speaking, if medical treatment is needed for a child with DSD, it will be a form of hormone replacement. Some children require sex hormone replacement to support their pubertal development or sexual maturation, as well as to maintain their adult reproductive anatomy and function. Other children require hormone replacement related to adrenal gland function or general growth and development. We review broad categories of hormone replacement commonly recommended for children with DSD in the sections below.

46,XX DSD Due to CAH

Children with CAH require daily replacement of the stress hormone cortisol to survive. Depending on the type of cortisol replacement prescribed, your son or daughter may take this medicine up to three times a day. If your child is ill or is having surgery, the dose needs to be increased to compensate for the associated stress. Many children with CAH take a second type of medicine (fludrocortisone or florinef) to replace the hormone aldosterone. If needed, this second type of hormone replacement is usually taken once a day. If the prescribed adrenal hormone replacement is both correct and diligently given to girls with CAH, then they will develop a normal feminizing puberty and maintain healthy female reproductive anatomy and function as they mature into adulthood without the need for additional hormone treatment.

Options for medical treatment of CAH are limited by the type of cortisol replacement prescribed. Oral hydrocortisone is usually taken three times a day. Dexamethasone lasts all day and consequently is only taken once daily, but some physicians avoid this form of cortisol replacement because it is highly potent. The keys to effective and safe cortisol replacement are frequent monitoring of growth and blood hormone levels and prompt medication adjustment when needed. Of course, as with all medications, you will want to check with your own health care team to determine the hormone treatment most appropriate for your child.

Girls with 46,XY DSD

Some girls affected by some forms of 46,XY DSD will have their gonads removed prior to puberty. Reasons for their removal are discussed later in the chapter. For these girls, estrogen replacement is needed at the age of puberty to promote breast development, overall sexual maturation, and optimal growth. If a uterus is present, combined estrogen and progesterone replacement can support normal menstruation. If sex hormone replacement is not taken by these girls at puberty, they will appear much younger than their age and their bone health will be compromised. Some girls with 46,XY DSD may also require other types of hormone replacement, depending on their diagnosis. For example, girls with adrenal insufficiency will need cortisol replacement.

A common concern about giving estrogens to young girls is that it might increase risk for breast cancer or other diseases common to women. It is important to remember that, in this case, estrogen is given to *replace* what would otherwise be present in healthy, developing girls. While risk for some medical conditions may increase with estrogen therapy, risk for other conditions will decrease (osteoporosis, for example). When we consider the overall effect of treating estrogen deficiency in girls with 46,XY DSD, health is enhanced, not diminished. Female sex hormone replacement is given as a pill or as a patch placed on the skin. The type of replacement will depend on your daughter's age and preference. You can discuss the options with your child's physician.

Boys with 46,XY DSD

Some boys with this form of DSD have a small penis at birth, with or without hypospadias (when the opening of the urethra is not at the tip of the penis). The penis size can be increased in most boys with 46,XY DSD by giving testosterone in infancy. Testosterone treatment may improve the outcome of future genital surgeries, if surgeries are part of your son's treatment plan. It is also thought that early testosterone treatment may lead to increased penis size in adulthood, but this is not proven. Early testosterone is typically given as three injections, 1 month apart.

Some, but not all, boys with 46,XY DSD will have their gonads removed prior to puberty for reasons that will be discussed later in the chapter. For these boys, testosterone is needed to support pubertal maturation and adult sexual function, as well as bone health. This later testosterone treatment is usually begun around the age of 12 or 13. Testosterone is either given as injections every 2 to 4 weeks or applied to the skin in the form of a patch or gel. All forms of testosterone delivery are effective; you and your son should discuss his options with his health care providers. Some boys may also need additional hormone therapy such as cortisol.

Girls and Boys with Sex Chromosome DSD

Girls affected by Turner syndrome and boys affected by Klinefelter syndrome usually require estrogen and testosterone replacement, respectively, to support and maintain pubertal development and bone health. This replacement is necessary even though the gonads are not typically removed in these children. It is also common for girls with Turner syndrome to take growth hormone to increase their overall growth.

Regardless of the type of DSD that affects your child, discuss with his or her health care team the need for hormone replacement therapy, including the benefits and risks associated with these treatments.

Surgical Treatment: Pros and Cons

As with medical treatment, surgical choices parents might consider are determined by the type of DSD that affects their child, as well as the gender of rearing of their child. Generally speaking, parents' surgical decisions fall under two major categories. The first is whether to proceed with gonadectomy (the surgical removal of the testes or ovaries) or genitoplasty (the surgical construction of female- or male-appearing external genitalia). The second is deciding at what age such surgeries should take place, if at all. For gonadectomy or genitoplasty, "early" means before 2 years of age, and "late" means after childhood. Below we will look at what happens during gonadectomy and genitoplasty, the typical ages for these procedures, and the advantages and disadvantages of having surgery versus choosing not to do so.

Gonadectomy: Yes or No? Early or Late?

Gonadectomy is usually done to prevent cancer by removing a cancer-prone gonad before tumors develop. Cancer of the gonads (testes and ovaries) can potentially develop in anyone. However, some people with DSD are at an increased risk of gonadal cancer. Gonadectomy is usually only considered in individuals with certain types of 46,XY DSD.

People with 46,XX DSD do not benefit from gonadectomy, because most have CAH with healthy ovaries that are not predisposed to developing cancer. Newborns with 46,XX DSD are usually reared female, and their ovaries support female pubertal maturation and reproductive function. In contrast, parents of children with 46,XY DSD may make decisions about whether (as well as when) to have their child's testes removed. Issues that should be considered before making important decisions about if, and when, to proceed with gonadectomy are discussed in the next few pages.

Girls with 46,XY DSD Who Are Unable to Produce Testicular Hormones

Some types of 46,XY DSD result in the complete or partial inability to produce testicular hormones such as testosterone and DHT and can result in a child having XY chromosomes and female-typical or ambiguous external genitalia. Some of these conditions are associated with an increased risk for developing testicular cancer. If this is true of your child, then your child's health care team may recommend early gonadectomy for your daughter.

Girls with 46,XY DSD Who Are Unable to Respond to Testicular Hormones

For girls with 46,XY DSD due to complete androgen insensitivity syndrome (CAIS), late gonadectomy is a reasonable option. Cancer of the gonads is rare (but can occur) before puberty in girls with CAIS, and there are advantages to leaving the testes in place until the girl is fully matured sexually. Pubertal development will occur without hormone supplementation because testosterone produced by the testes is converted to estrogen by the body, which in turn causes breast development. The natural hormones eliminate the need for taking medicine, which is an advantage because teenagers are not always good about taking medications consistently, partly because it makes them feel different. Another advantage of delaying gonadectomy in girls with CAIS is that the girl herself can have input into the decision when she is older. Nevertheless, estrogen replacement is safe and effective and works very well in girls who have gonadectomy prior to the age of puberty.

Gonadal cancer risk increases with age for women with CAIS; so women who retained their testes should consider gonadectomy once puberty is complete. For girls with 46,XY DSD as a result of partial androgen insensitivity syndrome (PAIS), the risk of testicular cancer is higher in this group compared with girls with CAIS. If the testes are located in the abdomen of girls with PAIS, gonadectomy upon diagnosis may be recommended. If the testes are located in the partially fused labia, the risk of cancer is thought to be lower.

Boys with 46,XY DSD Resulting from Problems with Testicular Hormone Production

Babies with 46,XY DSD who are completely unable to produce testicular hormones are typically raised as girls due to their normal female external genitalia. So, in this section we are only considering the issues concerning gonadectomy for boys affected by 46,XY DSD in whom there is a reduced, but not absent, production of testicular hormones. Some, but not all, of the types of DSD that affect these boys are associated with an elevated risk for developing testicular cancer.

Two kinds of 46,XY DSD that fall under the category "problems with testicular hormone production" require special mention because they are not considered to be at high risk for testicular cancer, and a near-normal masculinizing puberty is possible if the testes remain in the body. These special cases are 5α-reductase type 2 (5α-RD-2) deficiency and 17β-hydroxysteroid dehydrogenase-3 (17β-HSD-3) deficiency. In addition, some men with 5α-RD-2 deficiency whose testes have been left in place have been able to produce sperm.

There is a great deal of variability among the various diagnoses of 46,XY DSD in terms of the risk of developing testicular cancer, the ability to experience a masculinizing puberty, and fertility potential. Your son's doctors need to explain to you what your son's level of risk is, as well as his predicted puberty and fertility potential, before you make a decision about gonadectomy. If it is determined that gonadectomy is in your son's best interest, fertility will not be possible following surgical removal of the testes. However, testosterone replacement will be effective in masculinizing his body during adolescence and will support adult sexual function.

Boys with 46,XY DSD Resulting from Problems Responding to Testicular Hormones

In this section we consider the pros and cons of gonadectomy for boys affected by PAIS. In these boys, if the testes are located in a place other than in the scrotum (such as the abdomen), then the gonads are thought to be at higher risk for becoming cancerous, and early gonadectomy may be performed. When the testes are located in the scrotum, however, the risk for cancer is unknown. In that case, the doctors' recommendations may include biopsies and monitoring when the testes are left in place.

The benefit of gonadectomy for boys with PAIS is the elimination of the possibility of developing testicular cancer; a drawback is that boys who have their testes removed will be unable to produce their own testicular hormones or sperm. It is currently challenging, but not impossible, for men with PAIS who have not had gonadectomy to make sperm. If future advances in reproductive medicine improve fertility potential for men with PAIS, then the risks and benefits to early gonadectomy for this group will need to be reconsidered. In certain other conditions of limited male fertility, extraction of sperm from testes followed by in vitro fertilization has resulted in successful pregnancies.

The "Other" Group

If your child is affected by 45,X/46,XY DSD or 46,XX/46,XY DSD, then he or she may be at an increased risk for gonadal tumors, particularly if the gonads are located in the abdomen. For these children, early gonadectomy may be recommended. Children with ovotesticular DSD are usually raised female because they sometimes have fertility potential with their ovarian tissue.

In summary, when deciding on whether to proceed with gonadectomy for your child, several factors must be considered. For example, the risk of developing testicular cancer varies greatly from diagnosis to diagnosis, and as a result the benefit of early gonadectomy also varies. The effects of pubertal testicular hormone production are undesirable only for girls, and if the risk of cancer is low, removal of the testes can wait even in these girls until a time that best serves them. For some boys, there is a possibility for normal pubertal maturation or fertility if the testes remain in the body within the scrotum. The benefits of not proceeding with gonadectomy for these boys should be weighed against the boys' cancer risk. We encourage you to discuss the information provided here with your child's doctors so you and they can make the best decision for your son or daughter about proceeding with gonadectomy, as well as the best time to do so.

Genitoplasty: Yes or No? Early or Late?

Genitoplasty is a surgical procedure in which female or male external genitalia are constructed. Some, but not all, children with ambiguous external genitalia receive genitoplasty. We consider "early" genitoplasty to be surgery that is performed within the first 1 to 2 years of life. Late genitoplasty occurs around the time of puberty or later. Unlike gonadectomy, genitoplasty is not required to protect a child from serious health risks. However, many parents choose to proceed with early genitoplasty because they want to spare their children the teasing or embarrassment that they might experience due to their genital appearance or for technical reasons related to the planned surgery.

As with gonadectomy, sex of rearing is an important factor when parents make decisions about genitoplasty for their child with

DSD. The steps involved in feminizing genitoplasty for girls are (1) clitoroplasty (making an enlarged phallus look like a clitoris), (2) labioscrotal reduction (removing excess skin in the genitals to appear more feminine), and (3) vaginoplasty (the repositioning or creation of a vagina). For boys, the steps associated with masculinizing genitoplasty include (1) release of chordee (thin bands of skin that hold the penis in a curved position), (2) hypospadias repair (making the urine exit from the end of the penis), and (3) fusion of the labioscrotal folds (creation of a scrotum). Just as some parents decide not to proceed with gonadectomy, others decide to forgo early genitoplasty for their child, allowing the child at an older age to make his or her own decision about whether to proceed with these types of surgeries. It may not always be in the best interest of your child to have early genitoplasty.

We hope you will use the information in this chapter to help you understand your health care team's recommendations for proceeding (or not) with genitoplasty for your child with DSD. Parents should consult only with surgeons who are experienced in performing feminizing and masculinizing genitoplasty procedures.

Feminizing Genitoplasty for Girls with DSD

Feminizing genitoplasty is done with the goals of creating a female genital appearance, creating unobstructed urinary emptying and freeing the girl of incontinence or infections, and allowing for vaginal sexual and reproductive function. There are several surgical procedures for genital feminization. However, limited long-term outcome data regarding success rates for each procedure are available, and health care professionals disagree about the optimal timing for these procedures—about whether the results are best if they are done in infancy or later in adolescence or adulthood.

Clitoroplasty is the surgical reduction of an enlarged phallus. Clitoroplasty that preserves the glans (the tip) and nerves of the phallus is thought to result in better long-term sexual function than surgery that does not do so. While clitoroplasty can successfully make an enlarged phallus look like a clitoris, concern about reduced sensation and sexual responsiveness persists. While an enlarged phallus may place a girl with DSD at social risk for embarrassment or teasing, some parents defer decisions regarding clitoroplasty until their daughter is old enough to express her wishes about this type of treatment. Parents should take the time needed to weigh all the considerations of proceeding with this type of surgery for their daughter and should obtain a second opinion if they have any reservations about their decision.

Labioscrotal reduction is the surgical separation of fused labia and removal of excess skin that may have a wrinkled appearance that is more characteristic of a scrotum than of labial folds. This type of genitoplasty has not met with the same level of disagreement and concern that clitoroplasty has regarding if, when, or how to proceed. Often, girls will receive labioscrotal reduction at the time of clitoroplasty. Sometimes, tissue removed from an enlarged clitoris will be used to create the labia minora during labioscrotal surgery.

If you are considering labioscrotal reduction for your daughter, discuss the advantages and disadvantages of this procedure with her surgeon, including the best time to have the operation and whether it should be done at the same time as other procedures such as clitoroplasty.

In chapter 3, we described how your child's health care team might assess your child's internal reproductive structures. The results of these assessments will be extremely useful when deciding what type of vaginoplasty your daughter may need, if any at all. If your daughter has a vagina but its opening cannot be seen on the outside of her body, then vaginoplasty refers to *exteriorizing* the vagina or repositioning it so that it opens to the outside of the body. If your daughter has no vagina at all, then vaginoplasty refers to the creation of a vagina. When exteriorization is the goal, the type of vaginoplasty procedure used depends on the point of entry of the vagina into the urogenital sinus. When creation of a vagina is the goal, the type of procedure used may depend on the preference and experience of the surgeon performing the procedure.

Girls do not need to have a vagina prior to menstruation or having a sexual relationship that includes penetration. Why then do some surgeons recommend early vaginoplasty for girls? Often, when a girl is having early clitoroplasty or labioscrotal reduction, her surgeon will advise early vaginoplasty for two reasons. First, some surgeons believe that the surgical result is better in younger children because of improved healing. Second, some surgeons will use tissue collected during a clitoroplasty to create a vaginal opening, or "introitus." The use of this clitoral tissue is only possible if components of the genitoplasty are performed simultaneously. Surgeons who prefer early vaginoplasties may delay the procedure if no other genitoplasty is desired. When other surgeries such as clitoroplasty are chosen, then early vaginoplasty may be recommended.

When vaginoplasty is performed early, many girls will need additional procedures later in life, when they are ready to become sexually active, if they desire vaginal intercourse. The most common approach is to remove scar tissue that forms around the introitus. The advantages of waiting until adolescence or adulthood for vaginoplasty include the girl's ability to take part in her own medical decision making as well as decreasing the chance of significant scarring of the introitus. (Scarring is less likely to occur if a woman becomes sexually active soon after having the procedure.)

As with clitoroplasty and labioscrotal reduction, we encourage you to discuss the pros and cons of early versus late vaginoplasty with your daughter's health care team.

Prenatal treatment of CAH is a way in which medical therapy can be used to reduce or eliminate the need for genitoplasty in girls with CAH. It only applies to couples who know they might have a baby with CAH, that is, they have already had one child with CAH and are planning to have more children. For them, the chance of the next baby born having CAH is 1 in 4. Studies conducted several years ago showed that, in the case of CAH, masculinization of a baby girl's genitalia can be reduced or eliminated by giving her mother dexamethasone during the pregnancy. Dexamethasone is a form of cortisol that, when taken by a pregnant women, shuts off the excess androgen production by the fetus's adrenal glands. For the treatment to be effective, it needs to start very early in pregnancy (at or before 8 weeks). This is before one knows for certain whether that particular child needs the treatment. Even though there have been many mothers who have received dexamethasone throughout pregnancy, it is currently recommended that the treatment only be done as part of a research project. This is because we don't know enough about the long-term effects of dexamethasone exposure on children. See chapter 8 if you want more information about what is involved in research projects and experimental therapies.

Masculinizing Genitoplasty for Boys with DSD

Masculinizing genitoplasty is done with the goals of straightening the penis, placing the urethral meatus (urinary opening) as close to the tip of the penis as possible, and fusing the labioscrotal folds to more closely resemble a scrotum, if desired. For boys in whom the testes have been removed because of cancer risk, silicone prostheses that look and feel like testes can be placed in the scrotum. Taken together, these procedures will allow boys and men to have genitals that appear more male-like, to stand to urinate, and to achieve penetration during intercourse.

While it is not possible surgically to make a small penis bigger, testosterone treatment is commonly prescribed for boys prior to surgery to enlarge the penis. Additionally, the penis often appears longer once it is straightened following release of the chordee. In contrast to feminizing genitoplasty, there is currently less controversy regarding masculinizing genitoplasty. These procedures are frequently completed during the first year of life; there is little talk of "late hypospadias repair." Perhaps this is because the feminizing surgeries remove structures that cannot then be replaced at a future time if so desired, while masculinizing procedures build on anatomical structures that could be removed at a later date if the person with DSD so desires. Parents need to be aware that severe hypospadias often requires multiple surgeries to move the urethral opening near the tip of the penis and may be associated with problems such as scar tissue formation.

We encourage parents of boys with ambiguous genitalia to discuss the pros and cons of masculinizing genitoplasty with their son's health care team.

• *Chapter Summary* •

Medical and surgical treatment options for DSD vary by diagnosis and sex of rearing. We described some of the common medical and surgical treatment decisions that are considered by parents of children with DSD. Sometimes it is in the best interest of a child to have no treatment at all, while at other times action is warranted. This chapter is a guide to help parents work with their child's health care team to develop a medical and surgical plan that best serves their daughter or son.

• 6 •

Educating Children about DSD

Key Questions

Is my child healthy?
Why does my child need all these doctors?
Will my child grow up to look like other people?
Will my child grow up to behave like other people?

Many parents of sons and daughters with DSD avoid discussing their children's condition with them because parents want to protect them from potentially unsettling information. Because parents are unsure about how or when to talk about DSD, children may grow up with very little understanding of their bodies or of why they visit doctors. This lack of information can lead children to believe that there is something wrong with them. In this chapter, we provide suggestions on how to talk honestly about DSD with your child as he or she grows up. If you continue to talk openly with your child, your child will not only learn how to deal with this medical condition but will understand that there is nothing about his or her body to be ashamed of or to avoid talking about.

Is My Child Healthy?

Although most children with DSD are healthy, doctor visits can make children anxious about their physical condition. To ease some of the fear or discomfort that can surround such visits, we recommend assuring your child of health accomplishments when "teachable" moments present themselves. You can talk with your child at any time, but it may be particularly helpful to have a talk before and after your child's medical appointments. Talk to your child in an age-appropriate way to show that you are comfortable discussing body issues with them. For example, you might say, "I am so pleased with how much you've grown since school got out. I can't wait for Dr. A to see how tall you've gotten when we go to visit her next week." Or, if your child has successfully watched his or her weight, you could say, "The last time we visited Dr. B he was happy with how healthy you've been eating. I'm sure he will continue to be impressed with your snack choices when we visit him tomorrow afternoon."

After a doctor visit, you can congratulate children on how well they are taking care of themselves. For younger children, you might say, "When Dr. A checked your throat, I saw what a good job you are doing brushing your teeth. Keep up the great work!" For older children, you could say, "When Dr. B asked how school was going, I was proud of the way you answered him. You are really growing up." The goal is to focus on positive accomplishments, small or large, on a regular basis. Continuing to remind your child of his or her good health and the steps both of you are taking to stay healthy can be very rewarding in the long run.

It is also important for parents of children with certain life-threatening forms of DSD to offer reassurance and comfort (these conditions, described in chapter 3, include deficiencies in the adrenal glands' ability to produce hormones and problems with organ development). These parents might say, "I am so happy with how well you've remembered to take your medicine this month. It makes me feel good to see how healthy you are when you remember to take your pills." A parent may praise an older child by saying, "When I overheard you explaining why you had to miss school for your surgery, I was impressed with how knowledgeable you are about your health." By focusing on positive achievements, parents help their children realize that they—not DSD—control how they live their life.

If your family is fortunate enough to live in a place that offers support groups for people with DSD, these groups can provide a wonderful opportunity for you and your child to meet other individuals with this condition. Such experiences can have a profound impact on parents and children; it is inspiring to see other people with DSD succeeding in life and motivating others. If your hospital or town does not offer such opportunities, you might consider becoming active in national organizations (see chapter 9 for more information). Many of these organizations sponsor summer camps and regional meetings that facilitate peer support among children and families affected by DSD.

In summary, most children with DSD are healthy and, if your child is healthy, you should remind your child of this fact often. For children with life-threatening conditions, let them know that they can achieve and maintain good health by taking their medicine, visiting their doctors, and being informed. Finally, consider meeting with other people who are affected by DSD and who can offer your child additional support and reassurance.

Why Does My Child Need All These Doctors?

Just as important as assuring children about their health is explaining to them who their doctors are and why your child visits them. Again, by providing children with age-appropriate information, you will lessen their overall fear and anxiety. Let's start with how to explain the roles of certain members of your child's health care team—pediatric endocrinologists, pediatric urologists, and counselors (psychiatrists, psychologists, or social workers). Perhaps your child sees only a pediatric endocrinologist or perhaps his or her health care team includes other specialists not mentioned here. Consider modifying the following suggestions to meet your son's or daughter's circumstances and needs.

Visiting Pediatric Endocrinologists

To prepare young children (preschool) for a visit with a pediatric endocrinologist, first explain that these doctors help children grow up to be adults. Then explain that this is why these doctors measure how tall children are at every visit and keep a growth chart of each child's height and weight. After the examiner measures your child's height, praise your child for standing nicely and cooperating. Ask the endocrinologist to explain your child's growth curve and ask your child if he or she has any questions about growth. In this way you can encourage your child from a very young age to ask questions about why certain things happen during doctor visits. You also show your child that you support his or her active participation in these visits.

As children get older (5 to 7 years old), we recommend that you start explaining to them why their doctor examines their genitalia. You might begin by saying, "Do you know how boys become men and girls become women? This happens because of puberty. Your doctor checks your private parts to see that they are healthy and whether you are ready to start puberty." Most children between 5 and 7 years old can understand that boy and girl private parts are different and that all bodies are unique. We know that these talks can be intimidating to parents and children. When you talk to children about puberty or genital anatomy, they may act like they do not want to have this discussion with you. Avoidance is a normal reaction, which is why we recommend that you initiate these conversations with your child rather than waiting for him or her to ask you questions.

Before the endocrinologist does a genital exam, you might say to your child, "Remember we talked about puberty? Dr. A is going to check your pubertal development now and then we will ask her to explain to us what she sees." It may also help to give your child age-appropriate books that explain differences between boys and girls and how puberty happens. If you are uncertain what types of books to use, consult your pediatrician, local librarian, or online educational resources (available through the Sexuality Information and Education Council of the United States, www.siecus.org). Children can learn important information about their bodies by reading age-appropriate, scientifically accurate, educational material, even if they are too embarrassed to ask you questions directly. However, always assure your child that you will try to answer any questions he or she may have.

It might help *you* to remember that you are not the first parent faced with discussing genital anatomy and puberty with a child. We encourage you to seek and rely on the advice of others who have successfully accomplished this challenging task.

As children reach preadolescence and adolescence, their visits with endocrinologists will start to focus on how DSD influences fertility and sexuality. For adolescents who require hormone replacement to complete puberty, you can assure them that many people take hormones for this purpose. Praise your adolescent or teenager for remembering to take the hormones and encourage him or her to ask the pediatric endocrinologist about the pros and cons of taking these medications.

We recommend that parents provide older children and teenagers opportunities to speak with their pediatric endocrinologist without a parent present. In these situations, you might say, "I'm going to step out for a moment to check my phone messages. This is a good time for you to ask Dr. B or his nurse any private questions that you might have. When you're finished, join me outside and we can go to lunch." Giving children independence shows them that you respect their privacy and that you are in favor of them having honest discussions with their health care team as they move toward adulthood.

Visiting Pediatric Urologists

Many children with DSD will visit a urologist at some time. This might be because they are having problems with urinary tract infections or urinary incontinence or because they need special procedures that the urologist will perform. To prepare young children for such visits, explain that this doctor helps patients urinate or pee (depending on what word your family uses) without feeling pain or having accidents. Speaking with your child in an age-appropriate way will make him or her less afraid of the actual exam. If you are unsure about what will happen during an office visit, ask the urologist to explain exam procedures to you in advance (see chapter 3 for descriptions of some of the imaging tests a pediatric urologist might perform to define your child's internal urogenital anatomy).

Depending on your child's age and the type of test performed, the urologist may choose to use anesthesia. Again, we advise discussing what this means with your son or daughter ahead of time to reduce fear and anxiety. For example, you might say, "Dr. C is going to do a special test so she can look at where your pee comes out. That way she can tell us if this is why it has been hurting when you go to the potty. You will be given a medicine so it won't hurt at all and you won't remember it. After she examines you, we will know how to help you so that it can stop hurting." If the child seems anxious you can provide comfort and reassurance.

Frequently pediatric urologists are the specialists who perform genitoplasty on young children with DSD to make the external genitalia appear more male or female (chapter 5 describes the pros and cons of having these surgeries early in development). Regardless of whether your child underwent genitoplasty at an early age, help him or her understand that no two bodies are exactly alike and that differences are not a bad thing. For adolescents and adults who decide to proceed with genitoplasty, it is imperative that they understand what is involved with these surgeries and what the likely outcomes are in terms of cosmetic appearance and sexual function.

We recommend open, frank discussions between parents, physicians, and children who are old enough to participate. An older boy who is planning on having hypospadias surgery should know the likelihood of experiencing postsurgical complications, the anticipated cosmetic and functional outcomes of having surgery, and how his life will be affected if he does not proceed with the surgery. If a young woman requests clitoroplasty, she needs to understand the likely cosmetic result of that procedure and her chance of experiencing postsurgical complications, including the possibility of a reduction in clitoral sensitivity.

For girls who underwent vaginoplasty during infancy or early childhood, reopening of the vaginal entry, or "introitus," may be necessary at adolescence to allow for sexual intercourse. This procedure is necessary because scar tissue can develop around a vaginal introitus when that part of the body is not used after surgery. Preparing your daughter for this possibility is important so that she is not surprised by the need for this procedure as she matures.

Similar to visits with the pediatric endocrinologist, we encourage parents to give older children and teenagers privacy to discuss health questions with their pediatric urologist. This allows children to have important medical conversations concerning urination, menstruation, and sexual function—all topics that can be difficult to discuss in the presence of a parent or caregiver.

Visiting Counselors

Many people benefit from talking about issues related to DSD with a professional who does not provide direct medical or surgical care. Counselors can help parents adjust to the stresses associated with caring for a child with a chronic medical condition, and they can help children work through anxiety associated with taking medication or being admitted to the hospital. Should concerns about gender or sexuality develop for a child as he or she matures, a counselor can provide positive reinforcement. For example, counselors can explain to your son or daughter that a person is not defined by appearance and that the size and shape of breasts and genitals do not necessarily affect one's ability to experience a happy sex life. To locate an appropriate counselor, you should consult your child's health care team or members of DSD support groups and national organizations (chapter 9 has more information on these organizations).

Visiting a counselor does not mean that you or your child have to participate in intensive mental health therapy or that either of you is experiencing serious mental health problems. Some people prefer to visit with a counselor just once or twice a year, and others simply want to meet a counselor so they have this resource established for their family should the need arise in the future. Other parents and children prefer the atmosphere of peer support groups or conferences supported by national organizations rather than formal counseling sessions (see chapter 10). You know what is best for you and your child. We assure you that good counselors exist who are knowledgeable about DSD and, if you think you or your child might benefit from talking to one, we encourage you to give it a try.

When My Child Grows up Will He or She Look Like Other Boys and Girls?

In chapter 5, we described some of the medical treatments offered by pediatric endocrinologists to support growth and pubertal development in children and adolescents with DSD. We also described how pediatric urologists perform genitoplasty on some people so that their genitalia more closely resemble their gender of rearing. Depending on your child's type of DSD and the medical and surgical decisions that you have made, your son or daughter may look very much, or very little, like other boys and girls of a similar age.

Girls with 46,XX DSD due to CAH will grow pubic hair, develop breasts, and menstruate similarly to girls without DSD when treated appropriately with cortisol replacement. You can assure your daughter that if she remembers to take her pills every day, she will be like her female friends in terms of wearing a bra, having a pubertal growth spurt, and getting periods. Your daughter should also understand that she might become pregnant or acquire a sexually transmitted disease (STD) if she has unprotected sex—just like her friends who do not have CAH. If your daughter was born with moderate-to-severe masculinization of her genitalia, and if you opted not to proceed with feminizing genitoplasty during her infancy or childhood, then her genital anatomy will look different from that of her female friends. If your daughter received early feminizing surgery, then her genitalia will more closely resemble that of her friends; however, there may still be some differences.

Girls with 46,XY DSD will also develop breasts if they are exposed to estrogen (produced by their body or from hormone replacement administered as a patch or a pill) during puberty. Some girls will have little or no pubic hair and will not menstruate, depending on their specific type of 46,XY DSD. We encourage you to ask your daughter's pediatric endocrinologist what your daughter's pubertal development is likely to be so that your daughter can be told what she can expect during adolescence. Some girls with 46,XY DSD are born with genitals that look no different from those of girls without DSD, while others are born with ambiguous genitalia. The physical appearance of girls in the latter group will depend on whether or not they previously underwent genitoplasty. Although girls with 46,XY DSD will not get pregnant, they can catch STDs if they have unprotected sex. It is important to discuss safe sex practices with your daughter as she enters adolescence.

Boys with 46,XY DSD will grow and develop muscles and body hair as long as they are exposed to testosterone during puberty (either produced by their body or as a result of hormone replacement therapy administered as an intramuscular injection or rubbed onto the skin). Some boys will experience substantial growth of their penis during puberty, depending on the specific type of DSD that affects them. For boys whose testes were removed to avoid the development of cancer (as discussed in chapter 5), prosthetic testes can be inserted in the scrotum. If your son was born with undermasculinized genitalia, his genital anatomy will continue to look different from that of his male friends as he matures. This difference is usually most pronounced in boys who did not receive genitoplasty. Parents should discuss contraceptive options with their sons if they are fertile, but regardless of fertility, boys with 46,XY DSD can acquire STDs. We therefore recommend that all parents educate their sons about safe sex practices as they enter adolescence.

For boys and girls affected by DSD, some physical differences are likely to persist as they grow from childhood to adulthood. However, these differences are strongly influenced by the cause of your child's DSD and the medical and surgical decisions you make for them as they grow. By preparing your child for the physical changes that accompany puberty and providing the necessary knowledge to avoid unplanned pregnancies and exposure to STDs, you can remove the fear and uncertainty many children experience during puberty.

When My Child Grows up Will He or She Behave Like Other People?

Remind your child that people with DSD graduate from high school and college, fall in love, have careers, get married, own homes, and have children. Just like people who do not have DSD, some have a biological child and others adopt a child or marry someone who already has children. By discussing DSD with children early on in their development, you let them know that there is nothing shameful about their medical condition or body. Expecting children to be informed and responsible for their health lets them know that they are worthy and capable of living a full and happy life.

Discussing fertility with a child with DSD can cause particular anxiety for parents. Although some children have normal fertility potential, others may require future medical interventions for conception or may not be able to conceive at all. We believe that it is important for parents to be honest and to answer all of their child's questions about fertility in an age-appropriate manner. We also believe that parents should emphasize that there are many ways for a person with DSD to become a parent and that reproductive options in the future may be much more extensive than they are now. Educating children with DSD from a young age allows them to plan for how and when they might want to begin a family that includes children, be it through adoption or other means.

• *Chapter Summary* •

Parents can reduce children's fears of doctors and hospitals by assuring them that they are healthy, praising them for taking care of their bodies, and preparing them for the physiologic changes that will occur when they enter puberty. Educate your son or daughter about why he or she sees certain doctors, and support active participation in his or her own health care. First and last, let your child know that there is nothing shameful about his or her body. The best thing for your child is to be informed about DSD and about how to be a sexually responsible adult.

• 7 •

Long-term Health of People with DSD

Key Questions

Is life expectancy different for people with DSD?
Is my child at risk for other medical conditions because of DSD?
How will hormone replacement affect long-term health?

Most people with DSD live out their lives as healthy individuals. This is true even for those affected by life-threatening conditions, such as CAH, provided they receive appropriate education and medical therapy. In this chapter, we explore what is known about the life expectancy and long-term health of people with DSD.

Our understanding of the long-term health of people with DSD is incomplete for many reasons. In some cases, like in people with CAH, the initial research focused on the critical need for early cortisol treatment and how surgical procedures should be performed; only recently has attention been directed toward understanding the health of middle-aged or older adults with these conditions. Another explanation for our incomplete understanding is that many people with different forms of DSD stop visiting specialists after they reach adulthood. As a result, we have not learned enough about the natural history of DSD. Finally, some types of DSD are so uncommon that gathering meaningful data from individuals concerning their long-term health is simply going to take a long time.

Even though we wish there was more information about the

long-term health of people with different types of DSD, we still know a lot about what to expect based on experience with other conditions and on the wealth of information available on reproductive biology and health in the population as a whole.

Is Life Expectancy Different for People with DSD?

People with 46,XX DSD have the same life expectancy as individuals who don't have it. As long as they receive necessary medical treatment, such as cortisol and aldosterone replacement, even people with 46,XX DSD who do not produce adequate amounts of adrenal hormones will have the same life expectancy as that of the general population. For this group, DSD neither causes nor protects against earlier than normal mortality. The bottom line is that individuals with 46,XX DSD need to eat a healthy diet, exercise, and take required medications to maintain their health—just like everyone else.

For most men and women with 46,XY DSD, life expectancy is the same as for the general population. Similar to people who have 46,XX DSD, individuals with 46,XY DSD who do not produce adequate amounts of adrenal androgens can achieve and maintain good health when they receive appropriate medication. For people with 46,XY DSD and underdeveloped organs (most often the kidneys or heart), life expectancy can be lower than that of the general population. However, good medical care often results in long life spans for these men and women.

Klinefelter and Turner syndromes, two of the types of DSD categorized as "other," are associated with lower life expectancy than that of the general population. For men with Klinefelter syndrome, premature mortality can be caused by diseases that impact the cardiovascular, nervous, and respiratory systems. It is not known if increased mortality in men with Klinefelter syndrome is a result of genetic or hormonal aspects of their condition. In contrast, women with Turner syndrome experience premature mortality almost exclusively because of complications resulting from cardiovascular disease, such as defects of the aortic arch and valve. Hypertension is also commonly associated with Turner syndrome. Therefore, careful cardiovascular screening is recommended for this group of women throughout their lives, even in the absence of cardiovascular symptoms.

Is My Child at Risk for Other Medical Conditions Because of DSD?

When they get an unexpected diagnosis like DSD, many people worry about "what's coming next?" The fact that some types of DSDs increase your risk for additional problems or complications doesn't reduce this anxiety. However, consider this: knowing that other medical conditions might develop allows your doctors to monitor for them and then take steps early on to avoid serious problems. This is exactly the approach taken with DSD. These other medical conditions are all treatable, and the treatment is simplest and best when started early.

Cancer

In chapter 5, we discussed certain types of 46,XY DSD that are associated with the risk of developing cancer of the gonads (testes or underdeveloped gonads). Removal of cancer-prone gonadal tissue is recommended for people with particular medical conditions classified under the category of 46,XY DSD. In addition to cancer of the gonads, people with a specific type of 46,XY DSD known as Denys-Drash syndrome are at high risk for developing cancer of the kidneys early in life. If your child's health care team suspects that he or she may be affected by Denys-Drash syndrome, genetic tests are available to determine whether this is the case. Genetic testing can also help diagnose people with Frasier syndrome, a related type of 46,XY DSD. Frasier syndrome is associated with a high risk of developing a noncancerous type of kidney disease called glomerulonephropathy and with a risk of developing gonadal tumors.

Cardiovascular Disease

Women with Turner syndrome are at risk for cardiovascular disease throughout their lives. Consequently, regular cardiovascular screening is recommended, even for those without symptoms. The risk of developing type 2 diabetes mellitus, a medical condition that impacts cardiovascular health, is also higher in women with Turner syndrome. These women can protect themselves from developing this type of diabetes by eating a healthy diet, getting regular exercise, and maintaining a healthy body weight. For people with CAH due to 21-hydroxylase deficiency, conditions that impact cardiovascular health, such as high blood pressure, high cholesterol, and insulin insensitivity, are also common.

Other Endocrine Diseases

Women with Turner syndrome have an increased risk of developing hypothyroidism, celiac disease (a sensitivity to gluten that damages the small intestines), and diabetes mellitus. When detected and treated appropriately with diet or medications, these autoimmune diseases can be controlled.

Bone Disease

People with DSD who receive cortisol replacement for extended periods of time, such as those with CAH (46,XX DSD) or 46,XY DSD associated with adrenal insufficiency, can develop decreased bone mineral density (called osteoporosis) if their cortisol replacement dose is too high or is not closely monitored by a doctor. Similarly, people with DSD who do not make or respond to sufficient amounts of sex hormones (estrogen or testosterone) during puberty or adulthood have an increased risk of developing osteoporosis if they do not receive sex hormone replacement. For example, women with Turner syndrome have an increased risk of bone fractures when estrogen replacement is not initiated at an appropriate time or at a sufficient dose to support and maintain female pubertal maturation. Girls with 46,XY DSD as a result of androgen insensitivity syndrome require estrogen replacement at puberty to optimize their bone health if their testes have been removed. Some men with Klinefelter syndrome have decreased bone mineral density when their exposure to testosterone is suboptimal to support male pubertal maturation.

People with all types of DSD can take steps to optimize their bone health, such as making regular visits to the endocrinologist to ensure that doses of cortisol and sex hormone replacement are appropriate for their age, consuming adequate calcium and vitamin D, and maintaining appropriate levels of physical exercise.

Hearing Loss

Hearing loss is more common in girls and women with Turner syndrome than in the general population. Therefore, physicians need to closely monitor hearing in this group from childhood through adulthood.

How Will Hormone Replacement Affect Long-term Health?

Many individuals with DSD take hormones as replacement therapy. Most commonly these hormones are sex steroids (testosterone or estrogen), but sometimes physicians also prescribe adrenal hormones (cortisol) to people with DSD. You probably have heard that women taking oral contraceptives are at an increased risk of blood clots and certain cancers of the female reproductive system. You also may know someone who was treated with "steroids" for a disease such as rheumatoid arthritis and as a result became obese and developed osteoporosis. This kind of information may cause concern about the safety of taking long-term hormone replacement. Before we discuss some of these issues, remember that people with DSD take hormones to *restore* their body's chemical balance to levels that are appropriate for their age and gender. The benefits of hormone replacement clearly outweigh any risks of long-term side effects. Paying careful attention to the doses and forms of hormone replacement will minimize risks associated with these treatments.

Women with DSD who require estrogen (and progesterone in some cases) usually begin taking it when they are 11 or 12 years old and then continue it until the age of menopause, at which point they should discuss with their physician the pros and cons of continuing the treatment. During the course of their treatment, these women should have the routine evaluations (such as mammography) necessary to monitor their health.

For men and women with DSD who are taking cortisol, their doctor will make adjustments in their dosage as needed and may also monitor their bone health with special tests such as DEXA scans, which measure the calcium content of bones. In most cases, testing will confirm good bone health; if a problem is discovered, people with DSD can take specific steps to prevent major problems with bone health. The bottom line is that healthy people are meant to have specific levels of hormones in circulation at certain ages. Because some people with DSD cannot produce these hormones on their own, they should receive appropriate replacement therapy.

• *Chapter Summary* •

Most people with DSD have life expectancies similar to that of the general population. The few types of DSD that put people at risk for premature mortality are specific types of 46,XY DSD associated with an elevated cancer risk, such as Denys-Drash and Frasier syndromes, or cardiovascular disease such as with Turner or Klinefelter syndromes. Even for people with decreased life expectancy, attentive medical care can substantially lengthen life and decrease the chance of complications associated with having certain types of DSD. For these reasons, we encourage people to undergo careful monitoring throughout their lives by health care professionals who are experienced in treating people who have DSD. Over time, we will learn more about the natural history of these conditions.

· 8 ·

Challenges and Special Circumstances

Key Questions

Should I get a second opinion?
What if I want to change doctors?
What if I think my baby was assigned the wrong gender?
What if my child thinks he or she was assigned the wrong gender?
Should my child participate in a research study?

In this book we have explained what DSD is, how it occurs, and the medical and surgical options for treating aspects of DSD. We have also described how parents can educate their child about DSD, the child's pubertal maturation, and the likelihood of future fertility for a boy or girl with DSD. Our hope is that by being informed and knowing the medical options regarding DSD, parents will be better prepared to help their children understand the condition and to support them as they live and thrive into their adult years. In this chapter, we discuss unique circumstances that parents of children with DSD may face along the way and choices they might have to make. The title of this chapter reflects that not all families will experience these situations. Even so, all parents should be informed and be prepared to deal with them should they take place.

Should I Get a Second Opinion?

A second opinion involves taking your child to a different doctor to get another perspective on his or her health status and options for medical care. This doctor visit is also an opportunity to have a new person answer questions you have about your child's condition and treatment plan. Obtaining a second opinion does not necessarily mean that you are changing your child's health care provider; you are just gathering additional information and additional views. Second opinions for DSD can be valuable because medical and surgical treatment of these conditions is complicated. Because it's complicated, you need to be completely informed about the risks and benefits associated with various types of treatment decisions. We advise many parents to get a second opinion on their child's health care, so if you are asking the question, "Should I get a second opinion?" the answer almost always is "yes." Here we offer tips on how to make the most of a visit to a different doctor.

First, decide exactly what you want to get out of a second opinion. Do you have a specific question related to surgical, medical, or psychological treatment of DSD, or do you want a general assessment of your child's overall treatment plan? Making this distinction is important because it influences the decision about who is best to get a second opinion from. For example, if you have specific questions regarding options for a surgical procedure, then you would seek a qualified urologic surgeon or other surgical specialist for advice. If you want a broader evaluation of all aspects of your child's care, then review by a multidisciplinary team may be the best option.

After you decide you want a second opinion, we recommend that you ask for help from the doctors currently involved in your child's care. You might say, "I really appreciate your care of my child and how you've described the treatment plan for her. Before she has surgery, I'd like a second opinion. I would like your recommendations and suggestions as to where I might go for this."

Getting a second opinion should not damage the relationship you have with your current health care team. Second opinions are very common, and, given the complexity of DSD and its treatment, your child's doctors should understand your concerns and help facilitate your search. In addition to this, the doctor who provides a second opinion will need your child's medical records, and sometimes it is easier if the records are provided directly by your child's current health care team. Otherwise, you will need to obtain the records and carry them with you to the new doctor.

That said, you are not required to let your child's doctors know that you wish to obtain a second opinion; some people are more comfortable keeping this decision confidential. In addition, some parents might not want a second opinion from someone suggested by their child's current medical team. Perhaps they feel that by doing so, they would simply be referred to another doctor whose opinions about DSD would be the same. In this case, you might want to obtain names of doctors who can provide second opinions by contacting one of the support groups discussed in chapter 9. We suggest that the best option is to combine the two approaches by obtaining doctor names both from your child's current doctor *and* from support groups. If individuals or medical practices or programs are recommended by both, then you have probably located a physician who is qualified to provide a sound second opinion.

After you've decided on your specific goals in obtaining a second opinion and have selected a doctor, it is time to make an appointment for your child. The new doctor or team of health care providers will review your child's medical record, radiographs, and laboratory tests, take a personal medical history, and perform a physical examination. They will give their honest opinion about the status of your child's health and medical treatment, recommend any changes that they believe are indicated, and answer your questions. This process will be documented in their medical records, which you can keep for yourself or share with the doctors currently involved in your child's care. For many families, a second opinion is a one-time visit.

The bottom line on second opinions is that they are almost always worthwhile and should be pursued if you have questions regarding ongoing medical treatment. A second opinion gives parents a better understanding of their child's health care options, and it often makes them feel more comfortable with their child's current care. When opinions among doctors differ, you might choose to share the information from the second opinion with your current doctor. Your current doctor can review it and either make adjustments to your child's treatment plan or explain why he or she does not recommend doing so. If disagreement persists, you should go with the medical team with whom you are most comfortable, which might involve changing doctors. In the long run, you have made your child's interests and health your priority because you have made decisions with the best available information.

What If I Want to Change Doctors?

The diagnosis and treatment of DSD is serious and complex and can be very emotional. The care needed for your child is often lifelong, and opinions on treatment approaches can differ. For these reasons, your child's care is best accomplished when there is a trusting, respectful relationship among the medical team, your child, and other members of your family. However, this type of relationship is not guaranteed—or you might be comfortable for a time, but when circumstances change the comfort level might decrease. For example, sometimes parents are comfortable with a particular doctor, but as their child grows into adolescence, the child does not relate as well to the physician.

If you are unhappy with the medical care provided or the interpersonal aspects of your (or your child's) relationship with the health care team, what should you do? If your concern is about medical care, then you should consider a second opinion, as discussed previously. If interpersonal issues are standing in the way of optimal medical treatment of your child's DSD, then you might consider a change of doctors. For example, you might ask to see a different pediatric endocrinologist at your current medical institution. Or perhaps you will need to change medical centers altogether.

Although sometimes it's best to change doctors, that should be done only after careful thought and planning so that there is no interruption in your child's medical therapy. We suggest that you first carefully seek out physicians who can provide a second opinion (as described in the preceding section). After hearing their recommendations and getting a sense of how care would be provided by the new health care team, you may conclude that changing providers is in the best interest of your child. Be sure to tell your current doctor that your child is leaving the practice. He or she is still an advocate for your child's health and welfare and will be glad to know that you have found a good place for your child's future care.

What If I Think My Baby Was Assigned the Wrong Gender?

Health care teams should always include parents in decisions about gender assignment when a newborn's sex is unclear. If you think that you were not included in this important matter, you should consider finding a new doctor for your son or daughter. If you were included in your newborn's gender assignment but now question whether the correct choice was made, you should communicate your concerns to the health care team. You know your child best, and it is likely that you observe things about him or her that the doctors do not see during routine clinic visits. Additionally, your child will sense when you are uncomfortable or uncertain, even if you do not come out and explicitly voice your concerns, and it is possible that a parent's discomfort with a child's gender assignment can predispose that child to eventually question his or her own gender.

For parents who decide that their baby's initial gender assignment was incorrect, it is possible to change things. Generally speaking, the earlier gender reassignment happens in a child's life, the better. In the past, gender reassignments were not recommended for children older than 18 to 24 months of age. We now believe that 18 to 24 months may in fact be too late for some children; therefore, we encourage you to talk with your baby's doctors as soon as you suspect that an incorrect decision was made.

If you decide to proceed with gender reassignment for your baby, you will need to take several steps. First, you will have to change the stated sex on your baby's birth certificate (some states will require the use of an attorney). Second, if you decide to change your child's name, you must change it on all official records, such as medical charts and college savings accounts. Finally, you will need to educate family members and friends about your baby's gender reassignment. Concerning this last step, it is sometimes helpful to have a health care professional talk to your family and friends about why this decision was made. In our experience, when family and friends receive such an explanation and have an opportunity to ask questions, they rally behind parents to support the baby and the decision to reassign gender.

What If My Child Thinks He or She Was Assigned the Wrong Gender?

As we said earlier, it is generally not advisable to reassign gender in a child with DSD later than 18 to 24 months of age. An exception to this rule is when your child tells you that he or she does not identify with the assigned gender. Keep in mind (as described in chapter 4) that this is different from a boy who likes to play with dolls or a girl who is a "tomboy." In these instances, gender role may be atypical, but gender identity (that is, the gender that the child identifies with) often agrees with the child's gender of rearing.

If your child tells you that he or she does not identify with his or her gender of rearing, we recommend that you immediately notify your child's health care team. If the team includes a mental health professional who can assess your son's or daughter's gender identity, we encourage you to have this done. If you do not know someone who can perform such an assessment, ask your child's doctors to refer you to a qualified professional or consult members of national support groups for recommendations (see chapter 9).

After a mental health professional examines your child, any one of several outcomes is possible. It may be that your child's gender identity is *not* discordant with his or her gender of rearing, but that the child is simply exhibiting atypical gender role behaviors. When this is the case, you may choose to remind your family and friends that so-called atypical gender role behaviors are increasingly common in our culture and that this does not mean that your child's gender assignment was incorrect or should be changed. It is also a good idea to remind your child that differences in behavior between boys and girls, as well as among boys and girls, are substantial and contribute to making a person unique and valued.

It may also not be clear from a single psychological assessment whether your child is developing a conflict with gender identity. Perhaps your child is too young for a thorough evaluation or is not completely sure how he or she feels about gender identity. In these instances, it is best to have a psychologist or psychiatrist evaluate your son or daughter over a period of time until a clear picture emerges.

Another possible outcome is that a mental health professional confirms that your child does indeed have a conflict with his or her gender assignment. If this is the case, it will be necessary to revise your child's original medical treatment plan, including the support of pubertal development and genitoplasty (if applicable). You should explain to your child what will be different about his or her body after gender reassignment. You may also wish to update your child's birth certificate and legally change his or her name.

Most children who have undergone gender reassignment successfully live their lives according to the gender with which they feel most comfortable. A child who is transitioning to his or her new gender often feels tremendous relief, but parents and siblings may be unhappy with the gender reassignment. It is not uncommon for family members to mourn the loss of the child they were raising before the gender reassignment or for them to experience significant anxiety and guilt during the transition. For these reasons, we highly recommend counseling or support groups for children undergoing gender reassignment and for their families.

Should My Child Participate in a Research Study?

Research is essential for improving medical care of all people, including children with DSD. Decades ago, before we knew how to treat CAH, children were the first to try an experimental treatment, in the form of cortisone, for CAH; more recently, studies involving children taught physicians how to provide better treatment for people with CAH by using different medications and dosing regimens. As a result of those research studies, children with CAH receive far better medical care today than they did 50 years ago. Thus, if you are asked to enroll your child in a research study, carefully consider if this is a good option for you and your child. In this section, we provide more information about research studies to help you make such a decision.

Research involving people with DSD is usually designed to answer specific questions about the cause, natural history, or best treatment of these conditions. The intent is to find answers to questions about DSD and then publish the results so that other researchers and doctors can learn from them and patients can benefit from them. There may or may not be *direct* benefit to *your* child if he or she participates in research; it may be that the research will benefit other people eventually instead. Participation in a research trial is always voluntary; if you choose not to enroll your child, he or she will continue to receive the best possible medical care. If you decide to enroll your child in a research study, you ordinarily will be asked to sign a consent form that outlines your child's rights as a research participant and all that is involved in participating. There are many safeguards in place to protect your child's health while he or she participates in a research trial, but you are still the parent, and your judgment about how your child will react to participating in a trial is paramount.

Prenatal treatment of CAH (described in chapter 5) is an example of current research about DSD. This research involves a medication called dexamethasone that is used to decrease the masculinization of an infant girl's genitalia before birth. Such treatment may be beneficial because it reduces the need for genitoplasty in girls with CAH. However, because there is not yet enough information about the long-term safety and side effects of dexamethasone on babies exposed to the drug in the womb, the Endocrine Society currently recommends that physicians administer prenatal dexamethasone to pregnant women only as part of an approved research project. If you are considering participating in a research study like this one, take your time with your decision and make sure the investigators answer your questions. You need to be fully informed.

A therapeutic trial is different than a research trial. If your doctor wants your child to undergo a therapeutic trial, he or she believes that your child will benefit from a treatment that is not the standard care for your child's type of DSD. The new therapy might be a different form of a medication or the addition of a medication used successfully to treat other conditions. Usually there are published studies that show how effective and safe the treatment is for those other conditions. The intent of therapeutic trials is to provide the best care for an individual, not to gather data and publish results of a new treatment on a group of participants. There is no oversight by research ethics committees, and you won't be asked to sign a consent form. Your doctor will simply explain to you why it is worthwhile to try this treatment at this time and what is involved on your part.

• *Chapter Summary* •

Not all families of children with DSD will face the challenges that we have described in this chapter. However, all parents should be aware of the steps they can take to support their children through life's challenges. Obtaining a second opinion or changing doctors is your (and your child's) right, and we hope the information we have provided is helpful should you need to take this step. For parents of young babies with DSD, gender reassignment is possible, and we think that the earlier this is done, the better for the child and family. For older children, we do not recommend gender reassignment unless requested by the child and, in that case, an assessment from a mental health specialist is warranted before other steps are taken.

• 9 •

Peer Support

Key Questions

What can peer-support groups offer?
How do I find these groups?
How can I start my own peer-support group?

Participating in peer-support groups can help you learn about a medical condition and understand the risks and benefits of treatment. Peer-support groups may also increase your access to health care providers and help improve quality of life for you and your family. Because DSD is rare, it is unlikely that you know many people who are knowledgeable about this type of diagnosis and related treatments. In addition, you and your family may be sensitive about discussing sex and gender with other people, and you may feel isolated or alienated. Therefore, we encourage you to learn about support groups that help people affected by DSD. Once you do so, you can decide how large a role you want these groups to have in your life.

What Can Peer-Support Groups Offer?

As mentioned in chapters 6 and 8, peer-support groups can be an invaluable resource to you and your family in terms of education and physician referrals. By joining such a group, rather than dealing with DSD strictly on your own, you increase your self-confidence—you may feel better about your child's ability to live and thrive. Several people with DSD who we know have told us that before they met other individuals with similar conditions, they did not think that anyone else in the world had medical or treatment histories like their own. So, a peer-support group may be a good option for your child at adolescence or whenever he or she feels the need to meet with others facing the same concerns. When you meet other people with comparable medical experiences, you feel less alone and better equipped to face life's rewards and challenges.

Another important role for peer-support groups in the lives of people with DSD is to provide a confidential space where it is acceptable and comfortable to discuss feelings about DSD. Although family and friends offer support in their own way, they themselves have not lived with DSD. Members of peer-support groups will not be surprised by your thoughts and feelings, which means that when you participate in such groups, you will have the freedom to discuss your thoughts openly, without running the risk of censure or judgment from others. Talking with other individuals who have DSD or who are parenting a child with DSD reduces your feeling that no one else understands what you are going through.

How Do I Find These Groups?

National support groups for people with DSD are usually well organized. Phone numbers, email addresses, and websites put you in touch with these groups and lead to even more information. Many of these groups produce newsletters for their members and host annual conferences, as well. In table 9.1 we've included a list of such groups. Our list is by no means exhaustive; you can find information on other groups by searching the Internet or talking to members of your health care team. (You will want to be careful to check the credentials of any group you find on your own over the Internet. Ask your health care team for information.)

Although not a peer-support group per se, the ACCORD Alliance

Table 9.1. National Support Groups for People with DSD

Name of group	*Website*	*Membership focus*
AIS/DSD	www.aisdsd.org	Women and familes affected by any type of DSD
DSD families	www.dsdfamilies.org	Parents of children with DSD and teens with DSD
CARES Foundation	www.caresfoundation.org	Congenital adrenal hyperplasia
The Magic Foundation	www.magicfoundation.org	Various types of DSD
Turner Syndrome Society of the United States	www.turnersyndrome.org	Turner syndrome
The American Association for Klinefelter Syndrome Information and Support	www.aaksis.org	Klinefelter syndrome
Hypospadias and Epispadias Association	http://heainfo.org/index.html	Boys and men with various types of 46,XY DSD

(www.accordalliance.org) is an organization that is well connected with national and international support groups that serve people with DSD, and this group can make recommendations if you are seeking others for peer support.

How Can I Start My Own Peer-Support Group?

As a person with DSD or as a parent of a child with DSD, you may prefer to establish your own local support group rather than participate in larger, national organizations. Starting a peer-support group does not take any special training or certification—only the motivation and time needed to get the job done. If you plan on starting your own group, we encourage you to discuss this idea with leaders of national groups and health care providers in your area. These individuals can advertise your group to people in the local community and provide you with the necessary resources to get started. It is also a good idea to visit other groups in your area to see how they run. By talking with their members, you can borrow what works from these groups and avoid pitfalls that they have experienced. If possible, form an organizing committee that will share the responsibilities for starting and maintaining your group, and consider developing a website to advertise meetings and functions.

Before holding your first meeting, it is wise to consider some ground rules for how your peer-support group will function. For example, can family, friends, and health care professionals attend meetings, or will membership be limited to only individuals with DSD? After you define the membership criteria for the group, consider how to deal with confidentiality. Perhaps your members prefer to keep all information discussed within the group confidential or perhaps they will allow some level of discourse outside of the group as long as members are not identified to nonmembers. Whatever degree of confidentiality is decided on within the group, make sure that all members are aware of what is expected of them with respect to confidentiality.

The next step is to determine how often and where group meetings will take place. For example, group meetings associated with the SUCCEED Clinic in Oklahoma City generally take place on the evening of a clinic day, because this makes it possible for people who travel to Oklahoma City for their medical appointments to attend peer-support functions. If this plan appeals to you, ask your local health care providers about clustering clinic appointments for people with DSD on a common day, to make it possible for as many people as possible to participate in your group. You might also schedule some group meetings on weekends, to accommodate work and school schedules, and, if you live in a large state, you could consider alternating meeting locations in different parts of the state so the same people aren't always the ones to travel.

• *Chapter Summary* •

People with DSD often feel isolated, and they can be sensitive about discussing issues such as gender, sexuality, and fertility with others. You should know that you are not alone—many people with DSD thrive despite their diagnosis and treatment. A great way to meet other people with DSD is to become a member of a local or national peer-support group, or perhaps start your own group. Although initially it may be frightening to meet others and share your experiences, by doing so, you will feel less alone and will have the freedom to discuss your thoughts openly in a supportive environment. We hope that this chapter has convinced you that there is no reason to feel isolated by DSD. Other people with DSD can help you—and a great way to meet these people is through peer-support groups.

References

Chapter 1. An Introduction to DSD

Wiesemann C, Ude-Koeller S, Sinnecker GH, and Thyen U (2010). Ethical principles and recommendations for the medical management of differences of sex development (DSD)/intersex in children and adolescents. *European Journal of Pediatrics* 169: 671-679.

Lee PA, Houk CP, Ahmed SF, et al. (2006). Consensus statement on management of intersex disorders. *Pediatrics,* 118: e489-e500.

Chapter 2. What Type of DSD Does My Child Have?

Lee PA, Houk CP, Ahmed SF, et al. (2006). Consensus statement on management of intersex disorders. *Pediatrics,* 118: e489-e500.

Hsu CY, and Rivkees SA (2005). Congenital Adrenal Hyperplasia: A Parent's Guide. AuthorHouse, Bloomington, IN.

Congenital Adrenal Hyperplasia Research, Education & Support (CARES) Foundation at www.caresfoundation.org.

Major Aspects of Growth In Children (MAGIC) Foundation at www.magic foundation.org.

Chapter 4. Gender Development in DSD

Dessens AB, Slijper FM, and Drop SL (2005). Gender dysphoria and gender change in chromosomal females with congenital adrenal hyperplasia. *Archives of Sexual Behavior,* 34: 389-397.

Meyer-Bahlburg HF (2001). Gender and sexuality in classic congenital adrenal hyperplasia. *Endocrinology and Metabolism Clinics of North America,* 30: 155-171.

Lee PA, Houk CP, and Husmann DA (2010). Should male gender assignment be considered in the markedly virilized patient with 46,XX and congenital adrenal hyperplasia? *Journal of Urology,* 184: 1786-1792.

Chapter 7. Long-term Health of People with DSD

Bondy CA (2007). Care of girls and women with Turner Syndrome: A guideline of the Turner Syndrome Study Group. *Journal of Clinical Endocrinology and Metabolism,* 92: 10–25.

Chapter 8. Challenges and Special Circumstances

Lee PA, Houk CP, Ahmed SF, et al. (2006). Consensus statement on management of intersex disorders. *Pediatrics,* 118: e489–e500.

Index